THE
ULTRASOUND
HANDBOOK

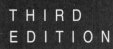

THIRD
EDITION

THE ULTRASOUND HANDBOOK

Clinical, Etiologic, and Pathologic Implications of Sonographic Findings

Rebecca Hall, PhD, RDMS

Director, Ob-Gyn Resident Ultrasound Program
Department of Obstetrics-Gynecology
University of New Mexico Health Sciences Center
Albuquerque, New Mexico

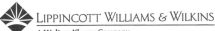

LIPPINCOTT WILLIAMS & WILKINS
A Wolters Kluwer Company
Philadelphia • Baltimore • New York • London
Buenos Aires • Hong Kong • Sydney • Tokyo

Acquisitions Editor: Lawrence McGrew
Editorial Assistant: Holly Chapman
Production Editor: Virginia Barishek
Senior Production Manager: Helen Ewan
Production Service: P.M. Gordon Associates
Compositor: Pine Tree Composition
Printer/Binder: R.R. Donnelley & Sons/Crawfordsville
Cover Designer: Deborah Lynam
Cover Printer: Lehigh Press

Third Edition

9 8 7 6 5 4 3 2 1

Library of Congress Cataloging-in-Publication Data

Hall, Rebecca
    The ultrasound handbook : clinical, etiologic, and pathologic
    implications of sonographic findings / Rebecca Hall.—3rd ed.
        p.   cm.
    Includes bibliographical references.
    ISBN 0–7817–1711–6
    1. Diagnosis, Ultrasonic—Handbooks, manuals, etc.   I. Title.
    [DNLM: 1. Ultrasonography handbooks.   WN 39 H178u 1999]
RC78.7.U4H35   1999
616.07′543—dc21
DNLM/DLC
for Library of Congress   98–40629
                                                            CIP

To Deborah,
my twin sister

PREFACE

In the past few years, the medical imaging community has been fortunate in seeing a vast choice of new material in each subspecialty become available. Diagnostic sonography has added Doppler and, more recently, Color Flow and Power Angio imaging to all specialty areas. There is now an explosion of new applications developing as a result. This new edition of *The Ultrasound Handbook*, in keeping with the concise summary format of the first two editions, includes brief comments about Doppler and Color Flow findings.

The purpose of this handbook is to give the imaging professional in diagnostic sonography concise baseline criteria for some of the more common pathologic conditions seen in this profession. Obviously, the many textbooks available supply greater detail on all aspects of these conditions. This handbook is not a textbook and is not meant to replace any textual material. Instead, it is meant to follow the volumes of material read by imagers as a source for concise review of etiologic, clinical, and sonographic information.

Imagers can carry *The Ultrasound Handbook* in their lab coat pocket when they are at their clinical sites and can quickly check findings expected for certain conditions when a textbook may not be accessible. The chart format provides a readable approach to each topic and allows space for personal notes.

Because so many professionals are entering the sonographic imaging field each year, including obstetric and radiology residents as well as diagnostic medical sonographers, this handbook has become a valuable review source for them. Although imaging resolution is improving, this handbook will remain a current source because sonographic findings are described in conventional sonographic imaging terms.

Rebecca Hall, Ph.D., R.D.M.S

CONTENTS

OBSTETRICS-GYNECOLOGY   135
OBSTETRICS   136

GYNECOLOGY 186

P R O S T A T E   211

R E T R O P E R I T O N E U M   217

T E S T E S   A N D
S C R O T U M   223

ABDOMEN

Echogenicity comparisons of major abdominal organs from least to most

renal cortex < liver ≤ spleen < pancreas < renal sinus < diaphragm

Normal gallbladder size

<10 cm length
<3 cm AP diameter
<3 mm wall

Normal liver size

<10–12 cm AP diameter at mid-clavicular line (transverse)
<17 cm superior to inferior length at maximum right lobe (sagittal)

Normal spleen size

<7 cm transverse width
<13 cm superior to inferior length (sagittal)

Normal pancreas size

<2.5 cm AP diameter (head)
<2 cm AP diameter (body)
<2 cm AP diameter (tail)

Normal adult kidney size

(Should note >1.5-cm difference between sizes of kidneys)
sagittal width: 9–12 cm
AP diameter: 3–4 cm
transverse width: 4–5 cm

Normal kidney echo pattern

Renal cortex is about one-third less echogenic than liver and spleen
Renal sinus is most echogenic
Medullary pyramids are most hypoechoic

Normal renal Doppler flowmetry

Renal artery peak systolic velocity is 100–120 cm/sec
Renal artery to aorta ratio (RAR) is about 2
Time to peak systolic velocity (acceleration time) is 1.0
RI <.70

ABDOMEN

DISEASE PROCESS	CLINICAL, LABORATORY, AND RELATED FINDINGS	ETIOLOGY	ULTRASOUND FINDINGS
ADRENALS			
Adenoma	Frequently nonhyperfunctioning, although most common cause of primary hyperaldosteronism (Conn's syndrome)	Arises from epithelium of adrenal cortex	Usually found incidentally
			May be bilateral
			Variable size, average 1–2 cm
	Can result in other endocrine abnormalities such as Cushing's syndrome		Usually appears as encapsulated, solid, uniformly hypoechoic lesion
			May have calcified components but is nonspecific
			May be multiple
Cyst	Usually asymptomatic	Rare	Usually found incidentally
	Patient may be hypertensive	May be result of hemorrhage into or around adrenal gland or of lymphangiomatous origin	Appears as anechoic lesion with strong back wall; posterior acoustic enhancement

DISEASE PROCESS	CLINICAL, LABORATORY, AND RELATED FINDINGS	ETIOLOGY	ULTRASOUND FINDINGS
		May be 2° to trauma	Characteristic posterior displacement of superior pole of kidney
		May be idiopathic	
			May calcify, in which case acoustic enhancement will be poor
			May hemorrhage, in which case cysts will not appear anechoic, but instead complex, primarily cystic, with internal echoes and posterior acoustic enhancement
Hemorrhage	Common in neonates	Birth trauma	Complex, primarily solid mass (depending on stage of bleed) anterosuperior to kidney
	Flank mass	Birth anoxia ▶	▶
	May have jaundice ▶		

DISEASE PROCESS	CLINICAL, LABORATORY, AND RELATED FINDINGS	ETIOLOGY	ULTRASOUND FINDINGS
Hemorrhage (CONTINUED)	May have ↑ bilirubin	Occurs due to high degree of vascularity of neonatal gland	Should decrease in size over course of weeks and resolve in 3–4 mos
	More common on right	Usually bilateral	Will displace kidney caudally and liver cephalically
	Will likely have normal levels of urinary catecholamines	In adults, most common cause is trauma	Won't see normal dense medullary core surrounded by hypoechoic cortex
		Usually unilateral	May eventually see calcifications (occur frequently following hemorrhage)
Metastasis	May be found incidentally	Metastatic extension 2° to often known history of lung, breast, or renal cancer or melanoma	Difficult to differentiate from adenoma
	Adrenal hormone function may or may not be compromised		Variable size
			Usually bilateral

DISEASE PROCESS	CLINICAL, LABORATORY, AND RELATED FINDINGS	ETIOLOGY	ULTRASOUND FINDINGS
			Solid, well circumscribed; totally encased within adrenal
			Overall picture is that of "headlight sign" (if bilateral)
			Central necrosis may occur in larger masses, leading to areas of decreased echogenicity within tumor
Myelolipoma	Usually asymptomatic	Rare	Highly echogenic adrenal lesion
	Patient may have pain due to hemorrhage, necrosis, or pressure on adjacent structures	Nonfunctioning tumor composed of fat and hematopoietic elements	May blend into adjacent perirenal fat when small
			Most are 2–9 cm in size
	CT and biopsy aid in further characterizing composition	Benign	Most are unilateral
			May see calcifications

DISEASE PROCESS	CLINICAL, LABORATORY, AND RELATED FINDINGS	ETIOLOGY	ULTRASOUND FINDINGS
Neuroblastoma	One of the most common intra-abdominal malignancies in children	Malignant tumor of neural crest origin	Heterogeneous, irregular solid mass
	May be asymptomatic	Generally arises within medulla, but may be of paravertebral, mediastinal, or retro-orbital origin	Calcifications commonly seen
	80% occur in children under 5 yrs; peak incidence between 2 mos and 2 yrs		Displaces kidney inferiorly rather than distorts it
		Widespread metastases occur early	May see retroperitoneal great vessel displacement
	Patient may: • Have failure to thrive • Be highly irritable • Have ↑ catecholamines • Be anemic • Have a fever		May see metastatic lesions within liver or, rarely, testes

DISEASE PROCESS	CLINICAL, LABORATORY, AND RELATED FINDINGS	ETIOLOGY	ULTRASOUND FINDINGS
Pheochromocytoma	May present with intermittent hypertensive episodes when BP is otherwise normal; associated with palpitations, headache, tachycardia, malaise, apprehension, excessive sweating	Arises from medulla, producing excess secretion of catecholamines	Tumors >2 cm in diameter; average size is 5–6 cm
		Usually benign	Seen as solid lesion with low-level echoes; well encapsulated
	May be asymptomatic	Hemorrhage and necrosis of tumor commonly occur	May occur extra-adrenally (10% of cases)
	↑ serum catecholamines		Usually unilateral
	May have ↑ urinary metabolites		Can be bilateral (10%)
			To appreciate origin, very careful attention to anatomic displacement is necessary (e.g., may displace IVC anteriorly)

DISEASE PROCESS	CLINICAL, LABORATORY, AND RELATED FINDINGS	ETIOLOGY	ULTRASOUND FINDINGS
ABDOMINAL AORTA			
Normal			Lumen generally <3 cm; specific size of normal lumen: • Proximal aorta, 2.3 cm • At renal arteries, 2 cm • Below renal arteries, 1.8 cm • At bifurcation, 1.5 cm • Iliac vessels, 1.0 cm
Ectatic	Asymptomatic	Degenerative changes in medial wall of vasculature	Color Doppler rapidly assesses arterial size, lumen size, and flow pattern Diffuse enlargement of aorta from diaphragm to bifurcation Normal AP measurement may be >3 cm

DISEASE PROCESS	CLINICAL, LABORATORY, AND RELATED FINDINGS	ETIOLOGY	ULTRASOUND FINDINGS
			May appear tortuous as artery progresses downward
Aneurysm	Occurs in up to 2% of general population	Degeneration and weakening of medial layer of artery	May be found incidentally
	More common in elderly men	Most often due to atherosclerotic changes in arterial wall	Dilatation of arterial wall >3 cm on AP measurement
	Ultrasound aneurysm measurements are consistently 1.3× smaller than those shown on radiographs	Trauma	Five measurement methods: • Anterior wall to posterior wall • Anterior wall to anterior spine (correlates with surgical and CT measurements) • Right to left diameter • Lumen size and measurement of thrombus thickness • Location within vessels

ABDOMEN

Aneurysm
(CONTINUED)

DISEASE PROCESS	CLINICAL, LABORATORY, AND RELATED FINDINGS	ETIOLOGY	ULTRASOUND FINDINGS
Dissecting	Patient usually known to have aneurysm	Intima is compromised; bleeding occurs between wall layers	May see intimal flap motion on real-time scan; pathognomonic for dissecting aneurysm
	Sudden onset of tearing pain	Associated most often with atherosclerosis	As blood volume increases, "double lumen" (false arterial lumen) appears
	Pain extends as dissection extends		Extends along length of vessel
	Patient develops shock		Color Doppler will demonstrate presence or absence of flow in both true and false lumens
Fusiform	Frequently asymptomatic	As above	Most common aneurysm type seen

DISEASE PROCESS	CLINICAL, LABORATORY, AND RELATED FINDINGS	ETIOLOGY	ULTRASOUND FINDINGS
	May be detected on routine exam as palpable, expansible mass in umbilical region		Uniform circumferential dilatation
			Usually below renal arteries
	Mild or severe abdominal or back pain		May see areas of increased echo reflections indicating thickening, calcification, and thrombi; may see acoustic shadowing
	Digestion difficulties		60% of the time, will see continuation of aneurysm to iliac arteries
			Color flow usually demonstrates turbulence

Graft

DISEASE PROCESS	CLINICAL, LABORATORY, AND RELATED FINDINGS	ETIOLOGY	ULTRASOUND FINDINGS
Leaking wall	May be asymptomatic	Repaired aortic aneurysm	As graft leaks, an anechoic perigraft fluid collection is seen along outer margins of graft; appearance considered abnormal after 3 mos postoperatively
	May see "ballooning" of skin surface, particularly if leak is in femoral portion of graft	Suture failure	Appears as false aneurysm—outer graft reflectors surrounded by irregular, variably echoic rim, depending on clotting setup
	Patient may experience severe pain		Color Doppler will demonstrate extraluminal flow or flow obstruction at any areas of stenosis or occlusion within lumen

DISEASE PROCESS	CLINICAL, LABORATORY, AND RELATED FINDINGS	ETIOLOGY	ULTRASOUND FINDINGS
Repair	None (postsurgery)	Repaired aortic aneurysm	Area of graft wall will appear sharply delineated and may appear ribbed
			Original vessel at each attachment appears slightly enlarged
			Graft may be placed within aortic lumen; will appear as two adjacent tubes traveling parallel to each other
Thrombus, intraluminal	Slowly progressive clinical manifestations (e.g., leg pain)	Formation of blood clot, usually occurring at site of an arterial atherosclerotic plaque or within an arterial aneurysm; worsens progressively as resistance to blood flow increases	Appears as low- to high-level echoes within the lumen
	Primary symptom is intermittent claudication that subsides with rest		Should appear in both planes ▶

DISEASE PROCESS	CLINICAL, LABORATORY, AND RELATED FINDINGS	ETIOLOGY	ULTRASOUND FINDINGS
Thrombus, intraluminal *(CONTINUED)*			More frequently seen along lateral and anterior than posterior walls
			May appear: • Anechoic (fresh bleed) • Complex with interfaces (clot with irregularities) • Hyperechoic (organized with vascularizaton)
			May appear as false lumen because of high-amplitude linear echo along wall surface of thrombus
			Color Doppler will demonstrate turbulent intraluminal flow and lack of flow at thrombus

DISEASE PROCESS	CLINICAL, LABORATORY, AND RELATED FINDINGS	ETIOLOGY	ULTRASOUND FINDINGS
APPENDIX			
Appendicitis	Most common cause of emergency laparotomy Acute patient presents with: • Vomiting • Fever • RLQ or periumbilical pain • Leukocytosis	Obstruction of appendiceal lumen followed by mucosal ulceration, abscess formation, and peritoneal involvement (if untreated)	Inflamed appendix appears as a noncompressible, aperistaltic, tubular, blind-ending structure Echogenic inner layer surrounded by outer hypoechoic layer measuring >6 mm in diameter May see highly echogenic focus within lumen (representing fecalith) If perforation occurs, may see heterogeneous, loculated pericecal fluid or free intraperitoneal fluid ▶

DISEASE PROCESS	CLINICAL, LABORATORY, AND RELATED FINDINGS	ETIOLOGY	ULTRASOUND FINDINGS
Appendicitis (CONTINUED)			↑ color flow, depending on degree of hyperemia in wall

GALLBLADDER/BILIARY TRACT

DISEASE PROCESS	CLINICAL, LABORATORY, AND RELATED FINDINGS	ETIOLOGY	ULTRASOUND FINDINGS
Carcinoma (gallbladder)	Most patients are in 60s–70s May be asymptomatic Dyspepsia Pain Jaundice Recent weight loss Advanced stage findings: • Inflammatory complications • Intestinal obstruction • Anemia	Rare; occurs in 2–3% of all cancers Types: • Adenocarcinoma • Undifferentiated carcinoma • Squamous cell carcinoma • Adenoepidermoid	Solid mass filling lumen of gallbladder; difficult to differentiate organ outline, most with intrinsic color flow Usually associated with stones (80%) Focal or diffuse wall thickening May see fluid levels representing necrosis

DISEASE PROCESS	CLINICAL, LABORATORY, AND RELATED FINDINGS	ETIOLOGY	ULTRASOUND FINDINGS
Cholecystitis			
Acute	Sudden onset of RUQ pain, especially postprandial; may be severe	Persistent obstruction of cystic duct by calculi	Gallbladder may be enlarged
		Bacterial infection within biliary tract	Gallbladder may have irregular outline and shape
	Pain may last for several hours or recur intermittently	Systemic infections such as hepatitis, AIDS	Thickened gallbladder wall, >3 mm
	Pain may radiate to back and right shoulder		Color Doppler may show ↑ wall and pericholecystic vascular flow
	Nausea, vomiting		May have anechoic striated area within wall due to pericholecystic edema (focal or overall)
	Fever		
	Profuse sweating		90% have cholelithiasis
	(+) sonographic Murphy's sign		▶
	Leukocytosis		

ABDOMEN

DISEASE PROCESS	CLINICAL, LABORATORY, AND RELATED FINDINGS	ETIOLOGY	ULTRASOUND FINDINGS
Cholecystitis, *Acute* *(CONTINUED)*			Presence of stones will fulfill sonographic criteria for Dx (see Cholelithiasis, p. 21)
Chronic	RUQ pain with history of intermittent similar pain	Usually due to nonacute intermittent presence of stones impacting cystic duct	Small gallbladder with thick, fibrous-appearing wall
	Nausea, vomiting		80% have cholelithiasis that fulfills sonographic criteria for diagnosis (see Cholelithiasis, p. 21)
	Severity of pain less than that of acute type (physical signs less marked)	Gallbladder mucosa inflamed and scarred, resulting in small, contracted gallbladder	
	History of vague dyspepsia, fat intolerance, and flatulence over long period of time		
	No significant lab findings		
Emphysematous	RUQ pain		
	Fever		

DISEASE PROCESS	CLINICAL, LABORATORY, AND RELATED FINDINGS	ETIOLOGY	ULTRASOUND FINDINGS
	Leukocytosis with shift to left	Form of acute cholecystitis with presence of gas-forming organisms in gallbladder wall or lumen (*E. coli* most common organism)	Irregular borders of gallbladder with echogenic gas and reverberation artifacts in gallbladder fossa
	May have slight increase in ALP, bilirubin		
	38% of patients are diabetics		May or may not be in association with stones
Gangrenous	No distinctive signs, symptoms, or lab findings to distinguish it from acute cholecystitis except pain more diffuse rather than RUQ	Mucosal ischemia in addition to severe, acute or chronic inflammation leads to hemorrhage, necrosis, and abscess formation	Gallbladder appears taut, with irregular lumen; ↑ color flow
			Will frequently see irregular striated thickening of gallbladder wall
			Commonly, pericholecystic fluid collections are seen

DISEASE PROCESS	CLINICAL, LABORATORY, AND RELATED FINDINGS	ETIOLOGY	ULTRASOUND FINDINGS
Choledochal cyst	Patient is usually <10 yrs of age Intermittent RUQ or abdominal pain May have palpable mass Jaundice May or may not have increased bilirubin	Congenital biliary tree anomaly of cystic duct, common hepatic duct, or common bile duct; results in obstruction of bile excretion; thought to occur as result of anomalous insertion of CBD into proximal pancreatic duct	May appear as focal fluid collection May appear as "second" gallbladder with dilated bile duct entering it May appear saccular or fusiform
Choledocholithiasis (common bile duct stones)	Jaundice occasionally seen Severe RUQ pain ↑ direct bilirubin ↑ ALP	Biliary obstruction distal to cystic duct as stone passes through CBD, most typically at the distal intrapancreatic portion	Dilated intrahepatic bile ducts (seen as parallel channels/"shotgun sign") proximal to stone May see actual stone within distal CBD with acoustic shadowing; may be difficult to see due to overlying gas

DISEASE PROCESS	CLINICAL, LABORATORY, AND RELATED FINDINGS	ETIOLOGY	ULTRASOUND FINDINGS
			Gallbladder size variable
			Stone likely to be visualized within gallbladder lumen
			CBD > 6 mm; CHD > 4 mm, although up to one-third of CBD calculi are found in nondilated bile ducts
Cholelithiasis	Patient may or may not be experiencing pain	Precipitates of one or more bile components; stone formation includes:	Echogenic foci within dependent portion of gallbladder lumen, which exhibit posterior acoustic shadowing
	If stone is in cystic duct, patient will likely be in acute pain either in RUQ or referred to left shoulder or chest	• Cholesterol	
		• Calcium bilirubinate	
		• Calcium carbonate	
	▶	▶	

DISEASE PROCESS	CLINICAL, LABORATORY, AND RELATED FINDINGS	ETIOLOGY	ULTRASOUND FINDINGS
Cholelithiasis *(CONTINUED)*	↑ bilirubin (although can be normal) ALP increases occasionally; AST, ALT likely normal unless liver cell damage exists	Posthepatic biliary cirrhosis 2° to congestive heart failure Due to: • Metabolic disturbances causing bile composition changes • Bile stasis • Gallbladder infection	Foci move to dependent gallbladder portion when patient position is changed Visualized echogenic foci with acoustic shadowing without gallbladder may occur if gallbladder is contracted or completely filled with stones
Common bile duct stricture	Jaundice Hx of cholecystectomy ↑ direct bilirubin ↑ ALP	CBD stenosis due to scarring	Tubular branching of dilated hepatic bile ducts (parallel channels or "shotgun sign") proximal to area of stenosis

DISEASE PROCESS	CLINICAL, LABORATORY, AND RELATED FINDINGS	ETIOLOGY	ULTRASOUND FINDINGS
			May see stenotic area at some point of CBD distal to dilated ducts
			CBD >6 mm proximal to the stenosis
			No porta hepatis masses seen
Empyema	History of acute cholecystitis	Extensive purulent inflammatory process due to untreated advanced cho ecystitis	Focal irregular gallbladder wall thickening
	Leukocytosis with left shift		Debris in gallbladder
	May have ↑ ALP		Pericholecystic fluid collection
Polyps	Patient may have RUQ pain	Most frequently cholesterolosis	
	May be asymptomatic		
	▶		

DISEASE PROCESS	CLINICAL, LABORATORY, AND RELATED FINDINGS	ETIOLOGY	ULTRASOUND FINDINGS
Polyps (*CONTINUED*)	No significant lab findings		Small, hyperechoic foci attached to inner gallbladder lumen wall; do not move to dependent portion of gallbladder but remain at same location even when patient moves
			Usually multiple; 2–10 mm
			No acoustic shadowing elicited by polyps
			May be on pedicle attached to wall
Sludge (gallbladder)	May be asymptomatic	Thick, inspissated bile most frequently due to bile stasis	Low-level homogeneous echoes layering dependent portion of gallbladder lumen
	Patient may experience intermittent RUQ discomfort		

DISEASE PROCESS	CLINICAL, LABORATORY, AND RELATED FINDINGS	ETIOLOGY	ULTRASOUND FINDINGS
	Patient may be in severe pain in conjunction with acute cholecystitis and/or stones	Result of patient being NPO, or in association with biliary ductal obstruction, pancreatitis, hyperalimentation	If patient position altered, sludge will slowly shift to next dependent portion of gallbladder
	Lab findings may be normal		Can form nonshadowing foci ("sludge balls")
	May have ↑ LFTs in association with changes due to obstruction		
KIDNEYS			
Abscess	Fever	Infection (hematogenous spread, urinary tract obstruction, or stasis) or bacterial reflux	Complex, primarily cystic focal lesion with echogenic debris and posterior acoustic enhancement; tends to alter renal morphology
	Chills		
	Localized tenderness		Irregular borders
	Occurs anytime		Thick walls
	Leukocytosis with left shift		▶
	▶		

DISEASE PROCESS	CLINICAL, LABORATORY, AND RELATED FINDINGS	ETIOLOGY	ULTRASOUND FINDINGS
Abscess (CONTINUED)	Patient may have anemia		Can contain septa
	Patient may have hematuria at onset		May see fluid-debris levels
			Little or no color flow
Acute tubular necrosis	Marked oliguria	Ischemia resulting from lack of blood supply to kidneys as a consequence of surgery, trauma, hypotension, heart failure, shock, etc., leading to necrosis of renal tubular epithelium	↑ kidney size, especially anteroposterior diameter
	↑ creatinine		Normal renal parenchyma
	↑ BUN		May see scalloping of renal sinus
	↓↓ GFR	Nephrotoxic injury resulting in necrosis of renal tubular epithelium	May see sharp delineation of swollen pyramids

DISEASE PROCESS	CLINICAL, LABORATORY, AND RELATED FINDINGS	ETIOLOGY	ULTRASOUND FINDINGS
Glomerulonephritis			
Acute	Variable	70% of cases result from immunologic response to exogenous agents such as:	↑ echogenicity of parenchymal cortex (only acute renal disease with ↑ echo pattern)
	Affects males more often than females	• Streptococcus (classic case)	Pyramids well visualized
	Usually affects young children and adults of any age	• Staphylococcus	Kidneys enlarged (bilaterally)
	Oliguria (<600 ml/day)	• Hepatitis B	With corrective treatment, kidneys revert to normal size
	Hematuria	• Measles	
	Hypertension	Other cases induced by:	
	Fatigue	• Glomerular basement membrane antibodies	
	Anorexia	• Tumors	
	Nausea/vomiting	• SLE	
	▶		

DISEASE PROCESS	CLINICAL, LABORATORY, AND RELATED FINDINGS	ETIOLOGY	ULTRASOUND FINDINGS
Glomerulonephritis, *Acute* *(CONTINUED)*	Sometimes fever		
	Edema		
	↓ GFR		
	Azotemia		
	↑ strep titers indicate recent strep infection		
	Hematuria		
	Leukocytosis with left shift		
	Mild proteinuria		
Chronic	Most common cause of chronic renal failure	Slow, progressive destruction of glomeruli from long-standing glomerulonephritis, causing tubule atrophy, interstitial fibrosis, and thickening of arterial walls	Grossly contracted kidneys (bilateral) due to loss of nephrons
	Insidious onset		Increased parenchymal cortical echogenicity compared to liver and spleen
	Eventual renal insufficiency variable at different stages		

DISEASE PROCESS	CLINICAL, LABORATORY, AND RELATED FINDINGS	ETIOLOGY	ULTRASOUND FINDINGS
	Oliguria		
	Polyuria		
	Hypertension		
	Proteinuria of varying degrees (50% of patients develop nephrotic syndrome)		
	Progressive azotemia		
Hematoma	Degree of ↓ hematocrit variable	Trauma	Focal lesion with complex, primarily cystic or solid components, depending on stage of bleeding process
	Trauma or hemorrhage in preexisting lesion (cyst, tumor, etc.)	Tumor	
	Mass may be palpable		Thick, irregular walls

ABDOMEN

30

DISEASE PROCESS	CLINICAL, LABORATORY, AND RELATED FINDINGS	ETIOLOGY	ULTRASOUND FINDINGS
Hydronephrosis	May be asymptomatic, especially if unilateral	Dilatation of renal pelvis and intrarenal collecting system, with obstruction of urinary flow due to:	Distortion of pelvocaliceal appearance: visualization of fluid-filled renal pelvis, calices, and infundibula
	May be found in conjunction with intermittent renal colic due to obstruction (e.g., calculi)	• Ureteral stones • Congenital anomalies of bladder neck, urethra, and ureteropelvic junction	Thickness of visible renal parenchyma is affected, depending on degree and length of hydronephrosis
	Patient may have hematuria if hydronephrosis is associated with calculi	• Pregnancy • Neoplasm	May be bilateral or unilateral, depending on point of obstruction
		Without obstruction, major causes include reflux, overhydration, diuretics, and overly full bladder	May see dilatation of the proximal ureter
		Chronic obstruction causes atrophy of the renal parenchyma	Must be seen before and after voiding in order to make ultrasound diagnosis

DISEASE PROCESS	CLINICAL, LABORATORY, AND RELATED FINDINGS	ETIOLOGY	ULTRASOUND FINDINGS
			Continuation after voiding indicates reflux
			May see bright, echogenic foci with acoustic shadowing at level of obstruction (calculus)
			Won't see dilated ureter with obstruction at ureteropelvic junction
			Color helps differentiate prominent renal vessels from hydronephrosis
			May see ↑ RI

KIDNEYS • Hydronephrosis

DISEASE PROCESS	CLINICAL, LABORATORY, AND RELATED FINDINGS	ETIOLOGY	ULTRASOUND FINDINGS
Leukemia			
Acute	Onset manifested by appearance of fever, progressive prostration, weakness, and malaise, progressing to hemorrhagic manifestations and bacterial infections; eventual hepatomegaly and splenomegaly	Malignant disorder of blood and blood-forming organs Basic cause unknown; environmental factors and genetic predisposition likely	Hepatomegaly Splenomegaly May see lymphadenopathy May see enlarged kidneys with echogenic cortex or focal poorly marginated mass with anechoic to low-level echogenicity; size returns to normal with chemotherapy
Chronic	Insidious onset, progressive weakness, weight loss, and lymphadenopathy; eventual hepatomegaly and splenomegaly Enlarged spleen, liver, and lymph nodes	Classification based on rapidity of disease and type of cell involved	Pelvic involvement may include lesions of testes, ovaries, and uterus May see secondary hydronephrosis

DISEASE PROCESS	CLINICAL, LABORATORY, AND RELATED FINDINGS	ETIOLOGY	ULTRASOUND FINDINGS
	Variable degres of anemia		
	Thrombocytopenia leads to bleeding		
	Leukocytosis leads to increased infections		
Lupus nephritis	Occurs primarily in females 20–40 yrs of age	SLE is an acute or chronic immune complex disorder that affects a patient's heart, vessels, kidneys, skin, lungs, lymphoid tissue, pericardial, and pleural surfaces	Increased cortical patterns
	Occurs in 70% of SLE patients		Kidneys may be enalrged or may appear normal, with normal corticomedullary differentiation
	Clinical manifestations include:	SLE causes circulating immune complexes containing autoantibodies to become trapped in glomeruli	
	• Arthralgia		
	• Vasculitis		
	• Renal disease		
	• Hematologic abnormalities		
	• Thrombocytopenia		
	• Anemia		
	• Leukopenia		

ABDOMEN

DISEASE PROCESS	CLINICAL, LABORATORY, AND RELATED FINDINGS	ETIOLOGY	ULTRASOUND FINDINGS
Lymphoma			
Hodgkin's	3:2 male-to-female ratio	Neoplastic disorder arising from lymphoid tissue with presence of distinct tumor giant cell (Reed-Steinberg cell)	Associated with hepatomegaly; parenchymal pattern may be normal or with diffuse, echogenic, infiltrative changes
	Primarily seen in young adults, aged 18–35 and after 45	Cause unknown, although genetic and viral origins theorized	Masses seen in spleen, liver, retroperitoneum, or testes are generally hypoechoic to anechoic; may displace adjacent organs or great vessels
	Patients present with:		
	• Nontender, rubbery, enlarged lymph node at cervical or clavicular area		
	• Fever of unknown origin		Lymphadenopathy may surround great vessels, creating a "mantle" appearance if diffusely enlarged
	• Dry, nonproductive cough 2° to higher lymphadenopathy		
	25% of patients >45 have mediastinal involvement		
	Adults >50 tend to have persistent fever, night sweats, weakness, malaise, weight loss		

DISEASE PROCESS	CLINICAL, LABORATORY, AND RELATED FINDINGS	ETIOLOGY	ULTRASOUND FINDINGS
	Lab values indicate: • Anemia • Leukocytosis		Kidney involvement: • Nonspecific, poorly marginated enlargement • Diffuse hypoechogenicity or focal low-level mass(es) with decreased acoustic enhancement Ultrasound differentials: • Abscess • Leukemia • Renal vein thrombosis • Acute pyelonephritis • Hypernephroma

KIDNEYS • *Lymphoma*

DISEASE PROCESS	CLINICAL, LABORATORY, AND RELATED FINDINGS	ETIOLOGY	ULTRASOUND FINDINGS
Lymphoma *(CONTINUED)*			
Non-Hodgkin's	Median patient age 50 yrs May be asymptomatic Patients present with: • Painless lymphadenopathy • Back pain • Fever • Night sweats • Weight loss Lab values: • Blood findings variable; may be normal at diagnosis to pancytopenia	Neoplastic disorder arising from lymphoid tissue; classification based on histologic type and behavior, including nodular and diffuse Unknown cause but immune mechanism theorized and viral mechanism thought to contribute to disease process Seen with increasing frequency in patients with AIDS and those who are immunosuppressed following organ transplantation	Associated with hepatosplenomegaly; parenchymal pattern may be normal or with diffuse, echogenic, infiltrative changes Masses seen in spleen, liver, retroperitoneum, or testes are generally hypoechoic to anechoic; may displace adjacent organs or great vessels. Lymphadenopathy may surround great vessels creating a "mantle" appearance if diffusely enlarged.

DISEASE PROCESS	CLINICAL, LABORATORY, AND RELATED FINDINGS	ETIOLOGY	ULTRASOUND FINDINGS
	• Abnormalities occur with advancing disease • Bone marrow affected early	Subsequent dissemination to bone marrow and other extranodal sites may occur	Kidney involvement: • Nonspecific, poorly marginated enlargement • Diffuse hypoechogenicity or focal low-level mass(es) with decreased posterior acoustic enhancement Ultrasound differentials: • Abscess • Leukemia • Renal vein thrombosis • Acute pyelonephritis • Hypernephroma

ABDOMEN

DISEASE PROCESS	CLINICAL, LABORATORY, AND RELATED FINDINGS	ETIOLOGY	ULTRASOUND FINDINGS
Masses, complex			
Multiloculated	Occurs in both children and adults	Rare	Involved cystic area is bulky; well-encapsulated cysts
	Presents with abdominal mass or abdominal pain	Nonhereditary	Septa
	Patient may have hypertension		Cysts sharply separated from surrounding tissue
	Patient may have hematuria		
Sinus lipomatosis	Usually occurs in obese patients	Fatty deposit buildup	Sinus may be hypo- or anechoic or ↑↑ echoes and thickened
	No significant lab findings	Benign	
Masses, cystic			
Caliceal diverticulum	Asymptomatic	Caliceal diverticula with calcium reabsorbed by tubules; unknown pathogenesis	Cystic area at calyx with bright, echogenic foci that may or may not shadow
	Found incidentally		
	Abdomen x-rays show calcification		May show movement of foci within dilated cavity

DISEASE PROCESS	CLINICAL, LABORATORY, AND RELATED FINDINGS	ETIOLOGY	ULTRASOUND FINDINGS
	Occasionally produces hematuria (due to hemorrhage)		Thin-walled, anechoic, smoothly contoured mass with posterior acoustic enhancement
	Rarely, produces hypertension		May see edge effect
	Most common renal mass		May have thin septations
	50% incidence in patients >50 yrs of age		
Hemorrhagic	Can occur in benign cysts	Trauma	Various stages of echogenicity from anechoic to complex, depending on age of bleed, clot, and resorption, with posterior acoustic enhancement
	Flank pain	Spontaneous rupture of cyst	
	Hematuria	Infection	Irregular borders
		Tumor	May see liquid-solid levels
Parapelvic		Uncertain etiology	
		▶	

KIDNEYS ● *Masses, cystic*

39

DISEASE PROCESS	CLINICAL, LABORATORY, AND RELATED FINDINGS	ETIOLOGY	ULTRASOUND FINDINGS
Masses, cystic, *Parapelvic* (CONTINUED)	Usually inferred from filling defect on IVP or found incidentally	Thought to be acquired lesions 2° to obstruction, with subsequent urine extravasation	Smooth-walled cystic mass with posterior acoustic enhancement
	May present as abdominal mass or UTI		Medially placed at renal sinus
	No significant lab findings		Displaces pelvocaliceal complex
			Calices don't communicate with mass
			No dilation of calices or ureters
Simple	Usually asymptomatic; discovered incidentally	Unknown cause	More commonly single but may be multiple; usually 1–5 cm but can become larger
		No inheritable tendency	
Masses, solid			
Adenoma	Asymptomatic	Metaplastic renal tubule lesion(s); may be solitary, multiple, or bilateral	Usually <3 cm
	No significant lab findings		Solid hypoechoic mass confined to the renal cortex
		Benign	

DISEASE PROCESS	CLINICAL, LABORATORY, AND RELATED FINDINGS	ETIOLOGY	ULTRASOUND FINDINGS
Angiomyolipoma	Occurs at any age, but mean age is 40 yrs	Proliferation of smooth muscle and blood vessels, with microaneurysms and various amounts of adipose tissue	Renal solid mass with ↑↑ echogenicity due to high vascularity and fat; usually unilateral; may be multiple
	Often occurs with tuberous sclerosis (80%) and then is usually asymptomatic	Benign	Focal, well-defined renal mass; tends to sit superior to renal sinus
	Frequently causes acute perirenal hematoma		Distorts renal architecture and parenchyma
	Hematuria		
	Usually affects females		
Carcinoma			
MESOBLASTIC NEPHROMA	Palpable abdominal mass	Most common renal neoplasm in first months of life	Solid mass
	↑ BUN		Coarse echogenicity
	↑ creatinine		Can be complex, primarily solid

KIDNEYS ● *Masses, solid*

41

DISEASE PROCESS	CLINICAL, LABORATORY, AND RELATED FINDINGS	ETIOLOGY	ULTRASOUND FINDINGS
Masses, solid, *Carcinoma* *(CONTINUED)*			
RENAL CELL (HYPERNEPHROMA)	More common in males over 40 yrs of age	Adenocarcinoma of functional parenchyma arising from tubular epithelium	Solid mass with irregular wall
	Anemia	Spreads via vascular system, lymphatics, adjacent organs	Can be hypoechoic, hyperechoic, complex, or isoechoic compared to cortex echo pattern
	Hypercalcemia	May cause perirenal hematoma	May have poorly visualized parenchymal interface or complex distorted appearance due to liquefactive necrosis
	Increased vascular blush on angiogram		
	Flank pain		May see metastatic extension into IVC, renal vein, or liver

DISEASE PROCESS	CLINICAL, LABORATORY, AND RELATED FINDINGS	ETIOLOGY	ULTRASOUND FINDINGS
	Hematuria		May see regional lymphadenopathy
	Patient may have no pain		
	Patient may or may not have fever		Color Doppler may demonstrate ↑ flow
	Metastasizes to lung, bones, brain		
TRANSITIONAL CELL	Affects males more frequently than females	Primary malignancy arises from renal sinus epithelium	Hypoechoic solid mass within renal sinus
	Patient may have colic hematuria		Ill-defined borders
	Flank pain		No acoustic shadow
	Gross hematuria		May see regional lymphadenopathy
	IVP filling defect implies tumor		
	40% 5-yr survival rate		Hydronephrosis may be 2° as mass effect

ABDOMEN

DISEASE PROCESS	CLINICAL, LABORATORY, AND RELATED FINDINGS	ETIOLOGY	ULTRASOUND FINDINGS
Masses, solid, *Carcinoma* *(CONTINUED)*			
WILMS' TUMOR (NEPHROBLASTOMA)	One of the most common malignant tumors of childhood	Malignant neoplasm arises within renal parenchyma	Large, predominantly solid, well-circumscribed intrarenal mass
	Peak incidence at 3 yrs of age		Variable echogenicity; complex pattern may show anechoic areas representing necrosis or hemorrhage
	Palpable abdominal mass		
	General malaise, weakness, failure to thrive		May displace pelvocaliceal system
	Hypertension (advanced stage of tumor)		May see metastatic extension to IVC, renal vein, liver, or peritoneal cavity
	Hematuria		
	Anemia (advanced stage of tumor)		May see lymphadenopathy
Nephrosclerosis	↑ blood pressure (>140/90)	Result of ↑↑ hypertension	Kidney may be normal or small

DISEASE PROCESS	CLINICAL, LABORATORY, AND RELATED FINDINGS	ETIOLOGY	ULTRASOUND FINDINGS
	Proteinuria	Results in narrowing of intrarenal vessels' lumina	Increased echo pattern of renal cortex
	Hematuria	May be benign or malignant	Parenchymal thinning
	↓ GFR		
	Benign: related to other manifestations of prolonged hypertension (e.g., heart disease, cerebrovascular accidents)		
	Malignant: cardiac complications, hypertensive retinopathy, neurologic complications, renal insufficiency		
Nephrotic syndrome	Edema	Primary glomerulonephritis	Enlarged kidneys
	Patient highly susceptible to infection ▶	Systemic disorder (e.g., diabetes, amyloidosis, renal vein thrombosis)	Hypoechoic or hyperechoic parenchymal cortex compared to normal

DISEASE PROCESS	CLINICAL, LABORATORY, AND RELATED FINDINGS	ETIOLOGY	ULTRASOUND FINDINGS
Nephrotic syndrome (*CONTINUED*)	Heavy proteinuria (>3 g/24 hrs)		
	Hypoalbuminemia		
	Hyperlipidemia		
	Lipiduria		
Polycystic kidney dysplasias			
Adult polycystic kidney disease	Patients in their teens or older	Autosomal dominant disorder	Bilaterally enlarged kidneys
	Affects both sexes	Formation of multiple cysts of kidney, spleen, liver, and pancreas	Parenchyma distorted by bilateral, ragged-looking cysts of various shapes and sizes
	Polyuria		May see associated cysts in liver (30% of cases), pancreas (10% of cases), or spleen (5% of cases)
	Hypertension		
	Hematuria		
	Proteinuria (50% of patients)		
	Azotemia		

DISEASE PROCESS	CLINICAL, LABORATORY, AND RELATED FINDINGS	ETIOLOGY	ULTRASOUND FINDINGS
	Flank pain due to mechanical distention of kidney wall by cysts		↑ resistive indices, especially in patients with hypertension
	Progresses to uremia		
Infantile polycystic kidney disease	Organomegaly	Autosomal recessive disorder	If in utero, see Obstetrics, Fetal Kidney Abnormalities
	Respiratory distress	Dilatation of collection tubules with little abnormality of nephrons	Bilaterally enlarged kidneys
	Hypertension		Hyperechoic cortex
	Cardiac failure	Associated with liver fibrosis	Hypoechoic liver
	↑ BUN		No "cysts" seen, but tiny cystic interfaces account for ↑ echoes
	↑ creatinine		
	Patients usually die within 2 yrs		
Multicystic dysplastic kidney disease	Flank mass		
	Hypertension		
	▶		

K I D N E Y S ● *Multicystic dysplastic kidney disease*

DISEASE PROCESS	CLINICAL, LABORATORY, AND RELATED FINDINGS	ETIOLOGY	ULTRASOUND FINDINGS
Polycystic kidney dysplasias, *Multicystic dysplastic kidney disease* (CONTINUED)	Nuclear medicine study will demonstrate no blood flow by lack of perfusion uptake	Dysplastic condition resulting from complete atresia at 8–10 weeks of the embryonal stage at the level of the pelvis and infundibulum or proximal ureter	Enlarged kidney(s) with many well-encapsulated, noncommunicating cysts that vary in size
		No familiar incidence	Random location within renal parenchyma
			Usually unilateral
			Contralateral kidney is usually normal
			Mav be bilateral (lethal)
Pyelonephritis			
Acute	90% of patients are female	Ascending bacterial infection of the renal parenchyma because of obstruction, stasis, reflux, or hematogenous spread; 80% of UTIs are from *E. coli*	Most common finding is normal exam
	Dysuria, frequency, urgency		

DISEASE PROCESS	CLINICAL, LABORATORY, AND RELATED FINDINGS	ETIOLOGY	ULTRASOUND FINDINGS
	Abrupt onset of: • Chills • Fever • Malaise • Back pain • Tenderness to palpation Leukocytosis with shift to left Leukocytic casts Pyuria Bacteruria	Less often: • Fungal • Viral	If unilateral, kidney is markedly enlarged, with decreased echogenicity of parenchymal cortex May have mild hydronephrosis May see focal hypoechoic area due to focal inflammation occupying entire wedge of kidney, with or without increased color flow
Chronic	Affects males and females Patient may be asymptomatic or may have insidious onset ▶	Recurrent UTI or inadequately treated acute pyelonephritis ▶	Contracted kidney Difficulty seeing renal borders Distortion of pelvis and calices ▶

DISEASE PROCESS	CLINICAL, LABORATORY, AND RELATED FINDINGS	ETIOLOGY	ULTRASOUND FINDINGS
Pyelonephritis, *Chronic* (*CONTINUED*)	Hx of recurrent childhood UTI	Chronic tubulointerstitial inflammation and renal scarring due to chronic obstruction or reflux nephropathy	Parenchymal thinning
	50% of patients have hypertension	May be unilateral or bilateral	Focal areas of ↑ cortical echoes adjacent to pyramids due to scarring
	Vague dysuria		
	Frequency		
	Polyuria		
	Nocturia		
	Pyuria		
	Leukocytic casts		
	Proteinuria		
	Intermittent bacteriuria		
	Azotemia		

DISEASE PROCESS	CLINICAL, LABORATORY, AND RELATED FINDINGS	ETIOLOGY	ULTRASOUND FINDINGS
	IVP may demonstrate clubbing of calices, irregular outline, thinning of cortical substance		
Xanthogranulomatous	May have poor or nonexcretion IVP contras	Result of chronic inflammatory process in an obstructed kidney	Focal or diffuse
	(+) urine culture for *P. mirabilis* or *E. coli*	Often associated with renal stones	Renal enlargement with multiple anechoic to hypoechoic areas
	Focal form can develop fistulae in renal parenchyma or GI tract		Shaggy borders
			Bright, dense central echoes with acoustic shadowing within renal pelvis
			Ultrasound differentials: • Can mimic renal cell carcinoma • Wilms' tumor in children • Renal tuberculosis

DISEASE PROCESS	CLINICAL, LABORATORY, AND RELATED FINDINGS	ETIOLOGY	ULTRASOUND FINDINGS
Renal failure			
Acute	Three stages:	A variety of diseases, drugs, and surgical procedures, as well as trauma, can cause:	Findings nonspecific
	First stage:	• Nephrotoxic injury	Kidneys normal in size or enlarged
	• Sudden oliguria (<400 ml/day)	• Obstruction	↑ parenchymal echogenicity compared to liver
	• Fluid retention	• Hypoperfusion	
	• Azotemia		Well-differentiated corticomedullary line
	• ↑ BUN		
	• ↑ creatinine		
	• ↑ WBC		
	• ↑ serum K		
	Second stage:		
	• Diuresis		
	• Dehydration		
	• Azotemia gradually disappears		
	• Normal BUN		
	• ↓ Serum K		

DISEASE PROCESS	CLINICAL, LABORATORY, AND RELATED FINDINGS	ETIOLOGY	ULTRASOUND FINDINGS
	Third stage: • Recovery • Anemia • GFR does not return completely to normal		
Chronic	Three stages: First stage: • ↓ of renal reserve • Asymptomatic • Normal lab values Second stage: • Renal insufficiency • Polyuria • Nocturia ▶ • Slightly ↑ BUN	Many different causes, including: • Infections • Inflammatory diseases • Hypertensive vascular disease • Connective tissue disorders • Congenital and hereditary disorders • Metabolic disorders • Toxic nephropathy • Obstructive nephropathy	First and second stages: • Decreased kidney size (bilaterally) • Parenchyma hyperechoic compared to liver Third stage: • Bilateral small kidneys (5–10 cm) • Shrunken renal parenchyma • Poor corticomedullary differentiation

ABDOMEN

DISEASE PROCESS	CLINICAL, LABORATORY, AND RELATED FINDINGS	ETIOLOGY	ULTRASOUND FINDINGS
Renal failure, *Chronic* *(CONTINUED)*	• GFR 25% of normal • Slightly ↑ creatinine Third stage: • Uremic syndrome (end-stage kidney disease) • Oliguria • Eventual complete derangement of excretory function • Multiple body system complications • GFR 10% of normal • ↑↑ BUN • ↑↑ creatinine • Fixed specific gravity of urine		
Renal vein thrombosis	Oliguria Hematuria	Thrombus blocks outflow, causing blood to engorge kidney	Enlarged kidney(s) May be unilateral or bilateral

DISEASE PROCESS	CLINICAL, LABORATORY, AND RELATED FINDINGS	ETIOLOGY	ULTRASOUND FINDINGS
	Proteinuria	Associated with metastasis, infection, trauma, maternal diabetes, dehydration	Diffuse, hypoechoic parenchymal pattern compared to normal
	↑ WBC		Color Doppler will demonstrate ↓ flow or lack of flow in distended renal vein to IVC and increased peripheral resistance
	Anemia		
Transplant			
Normal appearance	Kidney edema normal for 1–2 weeks	Renal failure leads to transplant	Use highest frequency possible
			Homogeneous cortex
Acute tubular necrosis	Common finding	Ischemia to tubules	Enlarged, swollen kidney (1–2 wks)
	Hypotension	Most common cause of acute posttransplant renal failure	Swollen pyramids
	Oliguria		▶
	↑ creatinine		
	▶		

DISEASE PROCESS	CLINICAL, LABORATORY, AND RELATED FINDINGS	ETIOLOGY	ULTRASOUND FINDINGS
Transplant, *Acute tubular necrosis* (*CONTINUED*)	↑ BUN Electrolytes altered		Parenchyma appears normal (not patchy, as in rejection) Doppler shows ↑ RI
Graft rupture	Can occur up to 2 wks postoperatively Abrupt onset of pain and shock Swelling over graft Anuria Urine leak (if ureter anastomosis separates) Hemorrhage (if renal vein or renal artery anastomosis separates)	Rupture of graft anastomosis	Gross distortion of graft contour Perinephric or paranephric anechoic fluid collection due to hematoma or urinoma Renal sinus of transplant may be splayed by possible ureteral obstruction and perinephric fluid collection
Lymphocele	Occurs 2–6 months postoperatively		

DISEASE PROCESS	CLINICAL, LABORATORY, AND RELATED FINDINGS	ETIOLOGY	ULTRASOUND FINDINGS
	Leg edema and tenderness	Severed or damaged lymph channels; lymph drains into retroperitoneal cavity to create fluid collection	Well-defined fluid collection separate from bladder or kidney
	Urine production maintained		Anechoic, with or without septa
	Painless swelling over the transplant		May see hydronephrosis
	No significant lab findings		Cannot differentiate appearance from that of urinoma
Obstruction	Oliguria or anuria	Stricture of ureterovesical junction	Splayed renal sinus due to obstruction and hydronephrosis
	No significant lab findings	Ureteral calculus	If calculus is the cause of obstruction, will see bright, echogenic foci with acoustic shadowing
		Abscess	
		Hematoma	
		Other stricture	Doppler: may see ↑ peripheral flow RI

DISEASE PROCESS	CLINICAL, LABORATORY, AND RELATED FINDINGS	ETIOLOGY	ULTRASOUND FINDINGS
Transplant *(CONTINUED)*			
Rejection ACUTE	Oliguria	Immunologic rejection results in congestion, edema, hemorrhage, or necrosis	Enlarged kidney
	Occurs within hours or up to years after transplant		Hyperechoic cortex
	Feeling of lassitude		Prominent, enlarged, anechoic pyramids
	Anorexia		Prominent collecting system
	↓ total urine output		Overall patchy parenchyma
	↑ creatinine		Indistinct corticomedullary boundary
	↑ BUN		Doppler reveals RI > 0.75
	Electrolytes altered		
	Nuclear medicine study shows ↓ perfusion uptake		

DISEASE PROCESS	CLINICAL, LABORATORY, AND RELATED FINDINGS	ETIOLOGY	ULTRASOUND FINDINGS
CHRONIC	Occurs up to several years after transplant	Gradual reduction in size of vessels due to arteritis	Kidney normal in size or small
	Progressive ↑ BUN		Irregular ↑ parenchymal echo patterns; difficult to differentiate parenchyma and renal sinus; Doppler shows ↑ RIs
	Progressive ↑ creatinine		
	Electrolytes altered		
Urinoma	Occurs 1–2 wks after transplant	Free urine collection from leak at ureterovesical anastomosis	Anechoic fluid collection; may be walled off or free
	Sudden oliguria		May form septa
	Fever		Cannot differentiate appearance from that of lymphocele
	Tenderness		

LIVER

Normal

Normal			Echogenicity of liver is medium level homogeneous

DISEASE PROCESS	CLINICAL, LABORATORY, AND RELATED FINDINGS	ETIOLOGY	ULTRASOUND FINDINGS
Abscess	Patient may have: • Localized pain • Fever • Chills • Anorexia • Jaundice	Usually pyogenic Bloodborne bacteria from direct extension of biliary tract because of surgery or trauma Pathogens usually polymicrobial	Complex mass containing septa and/or debris relating to pus, necrosis, or fluid; presence of gas with ↑ echogenicity and shadowing posteriorly
	↑ WBC	E. coli most common single pathogen	Irregular, thick borders
	Usually abnormal LFTs		Distorts normal parenchymal echo pattern
			May be difficult to see if located near diaphragm or if located peripherally, altering appearance of otherwise smooth border of diaphragm
Adenoma (hepatic)	May be asymptomatic	Benign epithelial tumor	Solid mass
			Well circumscribed

DISEASE PROCESS	CLINICAL, LABORATORY, AND RELATED FINDINGS	ETIOLOGY	ULTRASOUND FINDINGS
	May present with pain from sudden intraperitoneal hemorrhage	Rare, although increased incidence occurs in women taking birth control pills	Can be single (75%) or multiple (25%)
	Mass may be palpable	Creates increased vascularity, which can result in bleeding episodes	Usually appears hyperechoic, but appearance variable, especially if hemorrhagic
	No significant lab findings unless significant blood loss occurs		Size can range from small to very large (15 cm)
Cholangiocarcinoma	Intermittent jaundice is most common presenting symptom	Primary adenocarcinoma of bile duct epithelium	Intrahepatic bile duct dilatation appears as parallel channels/"shotgun sign"
	Pruritus	Originates in larger bile ducts; most often CHD or CBD	Extrahepatic biliary tree appears normal
	Mild, deep-seated upper abdominal pain		Usually no discrete intraductal mass visualized, although when seen, appears solid
	Weight loss		▶
	Nausea/vomiting		
	▶		

DISEASE PROCESS	CLINICAL, LABORATORY, AND RELATED FINDINGS	ETIOLOGY	ULTRASOUND FINDINGS
Cholangiocarcinoma *(CONTINUED)*	↑ direct bilirubin ↑ ALP Slightly ↑ AST Serum protein normal		May see distortion of porta hepatis Normal-sized gallbladder suggests upper duct involvement
Cirrhosis	May be asymptomatic • Hepatomegaly (although liver shrinks with advanced disease) • Splenomegaly • Ascites (increased abdominal girth) • Portal hypertension • Jaundice • GI bleeding • Decreased alertness	Progressive conversion of normal liver to abnormal nodules by diffuse fibrosis Common causes: • Alcohol abuse • Chronic viral hepatitis	Echogenicity of liver is much higher than that of kidney with ↑ attenuation; may be focal and patchy May see coarse echoes throughout diseased area due to fibrosis that may cause normal parenchyma to appear hypoechoic; color Doppler may show distorted and reduced intrahepatic vascular flow

DISEASE PROCESS	CLINICAL, LABORATORY, AND RELATED FINDINGS	ETIOLOGY	ULTRASOUND FINDINGS
	• Spider angiomata of face		Increased attenuation of sound due to fat; may cause difficulty in seeing far field of liver and diaphragm without utilizing lower MHz transducer
	• Palmar erythema		
	• Esophageal varices		
	• Weakness; muscle atrophy		
	↑ bili (serum and urine)		May see ascites
	↑ ALT, ↑ AST		May see splenomegaly
	↑ LDH		May see portosystemic venous collaterals; color Doppler detects reversed flow patterns
	ALP may be ↑		

Cysts

Echinococcus (hydatid)	RUQ pain with acute disease	Cyst stage of infection by parasitic tapeworm *Echinococcus granulosus*	
	Round, mobile epigastric or RUQ mass	▶	
	▶		

DISEASE PROCESS	CLINICAL, LABORATORY, AND RELATED FINDINGS	ETIOLOGY	ULTRASOUND FINDINGS
Cysts, *Echinococcus* *(hydatid)* *(CONTINUED)*	Hepatomegaly May cause increase in abdominal girth Percutaneous aspiration may not be performed due to theorized danger of anaphylactic reaction if viable larvae spilled into peritoneum	Endemic in major cattle- and sheep-raising regions ↑ incidence of disease in southwestern U.S., lower Mississippi Valley, Middle East, Australia, Mediterranean region, and Canada	Large cyst with thick, irregular walls and posterior acoustic enhancement typical of cystic lesions; may have low-level echoes (representing hydatid sand) May have adjacent "daughter" cysts, small to large, spherical to irregular, separated by normal liver tissue Walls may have calcific densities with acoustic shadowing
Multiple	May be asymptomatic May have palpable mass May have hepatomegaly		

DISEASE PROCESS	CLINICAL, LABORATORY, AND RELATED FINDINGS	ETIOLOGY	ULTRASOUND FINDINGS
	Usually normal LFTs May have minimal hepatocellular abnormalities	Usually associated with polycystic kidney disease (APKD), von Hippel–Lindau syndrome, or parasitic disease (see Echinococcus, p. 63)	Multiple variably sized, well-circumscribed, smooth-walled, anechoic lesions without color flow; posterior acoustic enhancement May also see cysts throughout pancreas, spleen, and kidneys
Simple	Occurs in 2½% of general population, increasing to 7% of population over 80 yrs of age Usually asymptomatic Hepatomegaly unusual Normal LFTs May have palpable mass	Usually idiopathic May be congenital Has an epithelial lining	Well-circumscribed, smooth, thin-walled, echo-free lesion measuring 1–20 cm Enhanced posterior acoustic transmission Multiple or solitary May see thin septa No color flow within cyst

ABDOMEN

DISEASE PROCESS	CLINICAL, LABORATORY, AND RELATED FINDINGS	ETIOLOGY	ULTRASOUND FINDINGS
Hemangioma	Occurs most commonly in women (5:1)	Most common benign liver tumor; contains vascular channels	Usually found incidentally
	Asymptomatic if less than 4 cm	Considered congenital rather than neoplastic	Most commonly echogenic but may have complex pattern; size varying from small (<3 cm) to giant cavernous hemangioma
	Larger lesions result in variety of presenting symptoms:	Benign	Serrated contour
	• RUQ pain	Tends to enlarge during pregnancy or with oral contraceptive use	Enhanced posterior acoustic transmission (occasionally)
	• Increasing abdominal fullness		Usually stabilize in size and echogenic pattern (may enlarge during pregnancy or when on BCP)
	• Anorexia		
	• Nausea and vomiting		
	No significant lab findings, except rare incidence of intraperitoneal bleeding		Color flow may show ↑ flow in tumor, but more often flow is negative
	↓ hematocrit may occur with intraperitoneal bleeding		
	Other LFT abnormalities, depending on severity and chronicity		

DISEASE PROCESS	CLINICAL, LABORATORY, AND RELATED FINDINGS	ETIOLOGY	ULTRASOUND FINDINGS
	Leukopenia		
Hematoma	RUQ pain	Blunt or penetrating trauma	Subcapsular or extracapsular, echogenic mass if acute; complex appearance after 24 hrs without color flow
	Large hematoma may result in ↓ hematocrit		Decreases in size as a result of lysis, leading to complete resorption or an anechoic mass
Hepatitis	Common liver systemic disease	Liver inflammation	*Acute*
	Clinical manifestations of different types are similar	Exposure to Type A, B, or C, viral hepatitis through fecal-oral, sexual, or parenteral route	Liver may appear normal or echogenicity may be diffusely decreased
	RUQ pain common	Other: alcoholism, toxins, drug reactions	Liver may appear enlarged, with normal echogenic prominent portal triads
	May have flu symptoms		▶
	▶		

DISEASE PROCESS	CLINICAL, LABORATORY, AND RELATED FINDINGS	ETIOLOGY	ULTRASOUND FINDINGS
Hepatitis *(CONTINUED)*	Loss of appetite (anorexia)		May see gallbladder wall thickening
	Nausea, vomiting		
	Fatigue		*Chronic*
	Jaundice, pruritus if severe		Hepatic parenchyma appears more coarse and inhomogeneous
	Marked ↑ AST, ↑ ALT (fall rapidly after several days)		
	↑ bilirubin		
Hepatoma (hepatocellular carcinoma)	Wide age group	Primary hepatocellular carcinoma (HCC) atypical parenchymal cells	Usually a discrete, single mass with ill-defined borders, but lesions may be multiple or diffuse
	Occurs more commonly in males (5:1)	Higher incidence in patients with cirrhosis (75%), following hepatitis, and in Asians	
	May have any or all of the following:		Appearance may be hyperechoic, hypoechoic, or isoechoic compared to normal liver parenchyma
	• Hx alcoholism		
	• Abdominal pain		
	• Palpable mass (RUQ)		

DISEASE PROCESS	CLINICAL, LABORATORY, AND RELATED FINDINGS	ETIOLOGY	ULTRASOUND FINDINGS
	• Hepatomegaly • Jaundice • Weight loss • Ascites • Splenomegaly Abnormal ALT, AST, protein, and prothrombin ↑ ALP and Bili if biliary obstruction (++) AFP in 50%		May see splenomegaly Color flow generally demonstrates increased vascularity surrounding and branching within tumor (75%) Metastasis to adjacent vessels appears as solid intravascular lesion with altered color flow
Leukemia			
Acute		Malignant disorder of blood and blood-forming organs ▶	Hepatomegaly Splenomegaly May see lymphadenopathy ▶

ABDOMEN

DISEASE PROCESS	CLINICAL, LABORATORY, AND RELATED FINDINGS	ETIOLOGY	ULTRASOUND FINDINGS
Leukemia, *Acute* *(CONTINUED)*	Onset manifested by appearance of fever, progressive prostration, weakness, and malaise, progressing to hemorrhagic manifestations and bacterial infections; eventual hepatomegaly and splenomegaly	Basic cause unknown; environmental factors and genetic predisposition likely	May see enlarged kidneys with echogenic cortex or focal poorly marginated mass with anechoic to low-level echogenicity; size returns to normal with chemotherapy
Chronic	Insidious onset, progressive weakness, weight loss, and lymphadenopathy; eventual hepatomegaly and splenomegaly	Classification based on rapidity of disease and type of cell involved	Pelvic involvement may include lesions of testes, ovaries, and uterus
	Enlarged spleen, liver, and lymph nodes		May see secondary hydronephrosis
	Variable degrees of anemia		
	Thrombocytopenia leads to bleeding		

DISEASE PROCESS	CLINICAL, LABORATORY, AND RELATED FINDINGS	ETIOLOGY	ULTRASOUND FINDINGS
	Leukocytosis leads to increased infections		
Lymphoma			
Hodgkin's	3:2 male-to-female ratio	Neoplastic disorder arising from lymphoid tissue with presence of distinct tumor giant cell (Reed-Steinberg cell)	Associated with hepatomegaly; parenchymal pattern may be normal or with diffuse, echogenic, infiltrative changes
	Primarily seen in young adults, aged 18–35 and after 45		
	Patients present with:	Cause unknown, although genetic and viral origins theorized	Masses seen in spleen, liver, retroperitoneum, or testes are generally hypoechoic to anechoic; may displace adjacent organs or great vessels
	• Nontender, rubbery, enlarged lymph node at cervical or clavicular area		
	• Fever of unknown origin		▶
	• Dry, nonproductive cough 2° to higher lymphadenopathy		
	▶		

DISEASE PROCESS	CLINICAL, LABORATORY, AND RELATED FINDINGS	ETIOLOGY	ULTRASOUND FINDINGS
Lymphoma, *Hodgkin's* *(CONTINUED)*	25% of patients >45 have mediastinal involvement Adults >50 tend to have persistent fever, night sweats, weakness, malaise, weight loss Lab values indicate: • Anemia • Leukocytosis		Lymphadenopathy may surround great vessels, creating a "mantle" appearance if diffusely enlarged Kidney involvement: • Nonspecific, poorly marginated enlargement • Diffuse hypoechogenicity or focal low-level mass(es) with decreased acoustic enhancement Ultrasound differentials: • Abscess • Leukemia • Renal vein thrombosis • Acute pyelonephritis • Hypernephroma

DISEASE PROCESS	CLINICAL, LABORATORY, AND RELATED FINDINGS	ETIOLOGY	ULTRASOUND FINDINGS
Non-Hodgkin's	Median patient age 50 yrs	Neoplastic disorder arising from lymphoid tissue; classification based on histologic type and behavior, including nodular and diffuse	Associated with hepatosplenomegaly; parenchymal pattern may be normal or with diffuse, echogenic, infiltrative changes
	May be asymptomatic		
	Patients present with:		
	• Painless lymphadenopathy	Unknown cause but immune mechanism theorized and viral mechanism thought to contribute to disease process	Masses seen in spleen, liver, retroperitoneum, or testes are generally hypoechoic to anechoic; may displace adjacent organs or great vessels.
	• Back pain		
	• Fever		
	• Night sweats		
	• Weight loss	Seen with increasing frequency in patients with AIDS and those who are immunosuppressed following organ transplantation	Lymphadenopathy may surround great vessels creating a "mantle" appearance if diffusely enlarged.
	Lab values:		
	• Blood findings variable; may be normal at diagnosis to pancytoma		
	• Abnormalities occur with advancing disease	Subsequent dissemination to bone marrow and other extranodal sites may occur	▶
	• Bone marrow affected early		

DISEASE PROCESS	CLINICAL, LABORATORY, AND RELATED FINDINGS	ETIOLOGY	ULTRASOUND FINDINGS
Lymphoma, *Non-Hodgkin's* *(CONTINUED)*			Kidney involvement: • Nonspecific, poorly marginated enlargement • Diffuse hypoechogenicity or focal low-level mass(es) with decreased acoustic enhancement Ultrasound differentials: • Abscess • Leukemia • Renal vein thrombosis • Acute pyelonephritis • Hypernephroma
Metastasis	May have known Hx of primary Ca May have any or all of the following:		Enlarged liver, diffusely abnormal appearance; multiple lesions likely with varied echogenicity

DISEASE PROCESS	CLINICAL, LABORATORY, AND RELATED FINDINGS	ETIOLOGY	ULTRASOUND FINDINGS
	• Hepatomegaly • Jaundice • Palpable mass • Weight loss • Splenomegaly • Ascites Abnormal hepatocellular function Increased ALP ↑ direct bilirubin	Most common liver solid mass is metastatic, most often 2° to adenocarcinoma colon; less often, 2° to breast, lung, pancreas, gallbladder, stomach cancer lymphoma, or melanoma	"Target" lesion appears as hypoechoic ring with echogenic center ("bull's eye"); color flow seen in 33% May see indirect finding of vascular displacement within liver Cystic lesions with irregular walls and acoustic enhancement due to necrosis may occur
PANCREAS			
Annular pancreas	More common in males ▶	Rare ▶	

ABDOMEN

DISEASE PROCESS	CLINICAL, LABORATORY, AND RELATED FINDINGS	ETIOLOGY	ULTRASOUND FINDINGS
Annular pancreas *(CONTINUED)*	Enlarged stomach and duodenal bulb Vomiting	Congenital anomaly occurring as a function of embryogenic development of ventral pancreatic bud, failure to migrate and fuse with dorsal bud, and subsequent envelopment around duodenum	Echogenic head of pancreas surrounds second portion of duodenum Echogenicity matches that of normal pancreatic tissue
Carcinoma	Broad spectrum of vague, nonspecific symptoms Painless jaundice may be a late symptom; may be accompanied by pruritus Recent weight loss; malaise 80% of patients may have dull to moderate midepigastric pain and malaise	Adenocarcinoma of pancreatic duct most typically arising in the region of the head (70%), 15–20% from body, 5% from tail	Typically a focal mass with complex, primarily solid, but hypoechoic echogenicity (depending on age of tumor) and irregular borders No intratumoral color flow usually seen Approximate measurement of mass is usually >2 cm

DISEASE PROCESS	CLINICAL, LABORATORY, AND RELATED FINDINGS	ETIOLOGY	ULTRASOUND FINDINGS
	May be asymptomatic		Enlarged pancreatic duct and/or CBD likely (due to extrinsic obstruction) with intrahepatic ductal dilation
	Appears more frequently in patients 50–80 yrs old; no high-risk population		
	Nausea and vomiting		In conjunction with enlarged CBD, may see taut, enlarged gallbladder (Courvosier's sign)
	May have palpable mass, hepatomegaly, or splenomegaly		
	0% 5-yr survival rate		May see ascites
	Tumors at head present earlier than at tail because of CBD obstruction		May see focal metastatic lesions in liver; para-aortic lymphadenopathy or porta hepatis
	↑ bilirubin		Ultrasound can be used to direct fine needle biopsy
	↑ ALP		
	↑ amylase		

PANCREAS ● *Carcinoma*

77

DISEASE PROCESS	CLINICAL, LABORATORY, AND RELATED FINDINGS	ETIOLOGY	ULTRASOUND FINDINGS
Cysts, true	No significant lab findings	Uncommon	Smooth borders
		Congenital or acquired; arise from within the pancreatic ducts and have an epithelial lining	Round configuration
			Variably sized
			May be single or multiple
Insulinoma	Variable; hypoglycemia and hyperinsulinism in 70% of cases; worsening of symptoms, including:	Most frequently occurring pancreatic tumor; β cell	Usually in tail or body
	• Palpable mass	Benign in 90% of cases	Appears hypoechoic
	• Sweating		Most are single; may be multiple
	• Insulin shock		Usually round or oval
	• Psychic disturbances		Most lesions measure 0.5–3.0 cm but can grow very large
	• Dizziness		
	• Nausea and vomiting		
Pancreatitis			
Acute			Pancreas often appears normal

DISEASE PROCESS	CLINICAL, LABORATORY, AND RELATED FINDINGS	ETIOLOGY	ULTRASOUND FINDINGS
	Restless patient with severe upper abdominal pain (corresponds roughly to region of inflammation)	*Adults* 90% are related to:	May see focal to diffuse enlargement
		• ETOH abuse	Distinct but irregular borders
	Patient usually has nausea and vomiting, abdominal distention, varying degrees of ileus	• Biliary tract disease (cholelithiasis most common)	Decreased echogenicity compared to normal (due to accumulation of fluid)
		Children	Extrapancreatic fluid collections:
	Patient may have pleural effusion	• Blunt trauma	• Lesser sac
		• Viral infections (such as mumps, measles)	• Anterior pararenal space
	Grey Turner's sign		• Perivascular areas
	↑ serum amylase		When resolved, pancreas reverts to normal echogenic pattern
	↑ serum lipase (subsides slower)		May see CBD stones
	↑ serum calcium (in severe cases)		

ABDOMEN

ABDOMEN

DISEASE PROCESS	CLINICAL, LABORATORY, AND RELATED FINDINGS	ETIOLOGY	ULTRASOUND FINDINGS
Pancreatitis *(CONTINUED)*			
Chronic	Begins insidiously but becomes constant epigastric and back pain with exacerbations	Associated primarily with chronic alcohol abuse and biliary tract disease; less often with ulcers, trauma, or metabolic disorders	Gland may be normal, smaller, or larger in size
	Aching distress rather than acute pain, becoming more and more progressive		May see focal enlargement with patchy groups of echoes
	May have mild recurrent jaundice		Irregular pancreatic outline
	May have nausea and vomiting		Dilatation and/or calcification of pancreatic duct may be seen
	Late manifestation is pancreatic insufficiency; diabetes develops		May identify calculi as small groups of dense echoes with or without acoustic shadowing
	↑ serum amylase (decreases with advanced chronic pancreatitis)		May see generalized decrease in pancreatic size with increased echogenicity due to fibrosis
	↑ serum lipase		

DISEASE PROCESS	CLINICAL, LABORATORY, AND RELATED FINDINGS	ETIOLOGY	ULTRASOUND FINDINGS
			Persistent on serial scans
Pseudocysts	Can be asymptomatic until adjacent organs are displaced or hemorrhage into cyst occurs	In children, due to blunt trauma	Walled-off fluid-filled mass lesions, either in or adjacent to pancreas
		In adults, usually due to acute or chronic pancreatitis	
			Irregular borders
	Persistent epigastric pain	Produced by pancreatic juice, edema, necrotic tissue, or blood, which becomes a sterile encapsulated fluid collection	May see anechoic or complex mass with or without dependent debris
	↑ amylase		
	↑ ALP if biliary obstruction develops from lesion	May fistulize, rupture, or become infected; may cause biliary obstruction	Enhanced posterior acoustic transmission
	May see calcifications on x-ray		May see displacement of adjacent organs or invasion of liver, lesser sac, stomach, left kidney, or spleen

▶

ABDOMEN

DISEASE PROCESS	CLINICAL, LABORATORY, AND RELATED FINDINGS	ETIOLOGY	ULTRASOUND FINDINGS
Pseudocysts *(CONTINUED)*			Can be found anywhere in abdomen
			Variable in size; can become very large
			May be confused with pancreatic cystadenoma
PYLORUS			
Hypertrophic pyloric stenosis	Infant previously healthy, with projectile, bile-free emesis; approximate age, 3–6 wks	Obstruction of the pyloric sphincter by sphincter muscle hypertrophy	Visualized best after water ingestion (60–100 ml)
	Repeated postfeeding vomiting	Precise cause unknown	Longitudinal pylorus >18 mm; pyloric muscle thickness ≥4 mm seen in both sagittal and transverse planes
	Dehydration		

DISEASE PROCESS	CLINICAL, LABORATORY, AND RELATED FINDINGS	ETIOLOGY	ULTRASOUND FINDINGS
	5:1 male:female ratio		Appears as echogenic central region (representing mucosa) surrounded by hypoechoic to anechoic ring (representing muscle)
	Palpation of olive-shaped, firm, muscular mass in RUQ		
SPLEEN			
Normal			Echogenicity of parenchyma similar to or may be slightly more than that of the liver; appears homogeneous except for vascular structures at hilum
Abscess	Pain (pleuritic or LUQ)	Trauma	May see mild splenomegaly
	Fever	Surgery	Difficult to distinguish from hematoma
	▶	▶	▶

DISEASE PROCESS	CLINICAL, LABORATORY, AND RELATED FINDINGS	ETIOLOGY	ULTRASOUND FINDINGS
Abscess *(CONTINUED)*	Leukocytosis	Altered immunosuppression mechanisms	Irregular borders
	Bacteremia		May see septa
	Septicemia		Complex fluid collection (internal echoes)
			May see pleural effusion
			Not confined to tissue planes
			May show reverberations associated with gas
Accessory	Occurs in 10% of popoulation	Normal variant	Area of echogenic tissue isoechoic to spleen
	No significant lab findings		Commonly occurs near hilum or pancreatic tail
			May be difficult to demonstrate if away from hilum

DISEASE PROCESS	CLINICAL, LABORATORY, AND RELATED FINDINGS	ETIOLOGY	ULTRASOUND FINDINGS
Asplenia	Asymptomatic	Rare	Nonvisualization of spleen
	No significant lab findings	Congenital	Liver more midline
	Nuclear medicine study is definitive modality for Dx	Associated with microgastria	
Cyst			
Epidermoid	Typically asymptomatic	Congenital; has epithelial lining	Large (10–15 cm), solitary, anechoic lesion
	Young patient		May compress surrounding organs if it becomes large enough
	May present with LUQ pain (due to complications such as hemorrhage)		May have internal echoes due to internal hemorrhage or infection
	No significant lab findings		Posterior acoustic enhancement

DISEASE PROCESS	CLINICAL, LABORATORY, AND RELATED FINDINGS	ETIOLOGY	ULTRASOUND FINDINGS
Cyst (CONTINUED)			
Hemorrhagic	Pain (LUQ)	Trauma (e.g. crushing injury or severe blow)	Subcapsular lesion appears as anechoic mass enveloping splenic parenchyma and conforming to splenic contour; pericapsular tear demonstrates free fluid surrounding spleen in LUQ or within peritoneal cavity; may appear complex, with ragged borders; low-level echoes within lesion, depending on stage of resorption
	Patient may be in hemorrhagic shock		
	Patient may have decreased hematocrit		Most will decrease in size over time and will resolve in weeks to months

DISEASE PROCESS	CLINICAL, LABORATORY, AND RELATED FINDINGS	ETIOLOGY	ULTRASOUND FINDINGS
Simple	Asymptomatic	Rare hydatid cyst (parasitic)	Echo-free lesions, usually solitary, surrounded by splenic parenchyma
	No significant lab findings	Unresolved hematoma	
		Trauma	May be found in conjunction with splenomegaly
		Cystic neoplasm	Well-defined borders
			Enhanced posterior acoustic transmission
			May compress surrounding organs it if becomes large enough
			If parasitic, may see dominant cyst with adjacent smaller cysts

DISEASE PROCESS	CLINICAL, LABORATORY, AND RELATED FINDINGS	ETIOLOGY	ULTRASOUND FINDINGS
Granulomatous inflammatory calcifications	Asymptomatic	Reactive hyperplasia	Usually found incidentally
	Calcifications appear on x-ray	Secondary to previous infection (acute or chronic)	Diffuse, punctate, echogenic foci may or may not show acoustic shadowing
Infarct	May be found incidentally	Sickle-cell anemia	Well demarcated
	May be associated with splenic pain	Malignant metastases	Wedge-shaped, hypoechoic area with base toward organ periphery
	Changes in lab values related to primary disease and its stage	Hypotension or occluded splenic vascular supply leading to global infarct	Spleen may atrophy, and echogenicity of lesions may increase over time
Metastasis	Variable, depending on type and stage of primary	Metastatic spread from primary malignancy, most often melanoma, breast, lung, ovary, and stomach	Discrete, solid mass usually hypoechoic but may have mixed echogenic pattern

DISEASE PROCESS	CLINICAL, LABORATORY, AND RELATED FINDINGS	ETIOLOGY	ULTRASOUND FINDINGS
			May be multiple
			May be complex, primarily cystic, due to necrosis
Rupture	Pain due to trauma or spontaneous rupture of enlarged spleen	Crushing injury or severe blunt trauma	Resembles hematoma
	Hematocrit decreased	Infectious mononucleosis, leukemia, malaria, typhoid fever, other types of acute splenitis	If patient has enlarged spleen without signs of organized hematoma, serial scans may show evidence of further enlargement
			With capsular tear, may see left subphrenic fluid
Splenomegaly	Clinically enlarged spleen or LUQ mass in conjunction with other disease manifestations ▶	Trauma	Most common spleen abnormality ▶
		Neoplasm (e.g., leukemia) ▶	

ABDOMEN

DISEASE PROCESS	CLINICAL, LABORATORY, AND RELATED FINDINGS	ETIOLOGY	ULTRASOUND FINDINGS
Splenomegaly *(CONTINUED)*	Other findings depend on etiology	Congestion (e.g., portal hypertension, cirrhosis, portal vein thrombosis, or stenosis)	Long axis >13 cm
			May see ↑ echoes of liver due to cirrhosis
		Systemic infections (e.g., AIDS)	May see ↑ PV, SV size due to portal hypertension
		Blood disorders (e.g. hemolytic anemia)	Color Doppler may show reversed flow in SV, PVs (hepatofugal flow)

BREAST

DISEASE PROCESS	CLINICAL, LABORATORY, AND RELATED FINDINGS	ETIOLOGY	ULTRASOUND FINDINGS
Normal	Ultrasound is most complimentary imaging modality when glandular, radiographically dense breasts are examined		Three echogenic components are seen sonographically: • Hypoechoic with low-level speckle-type echogenicities that represent fat • Echogenic reflective surfaces representing the connective fibrous Cooper's ligaments and fascial planes—the highest echogenicity within the breast tissue • Homogeneous medium-level echoes representing parenchymal tissue
	Mammography best in fatty tissue as fatty replacement extends into central core		Ducts are usually less than 2 mm

DISEASE PROCESS	CLINICAL, LABORATORY, AND RELATED FINDINGS	ETIOLOGY	ULTRASOUND FINDINGS
			Microcalcifications are not always visualized; when seen are not necessarily related only to malignancy
Abscess	Swelling	Inflammatory disease (mastitis)	Variable appearance, depending on stage of inflammation
	Pain	Occurs most commonly in the retroareolar region	
	Erythema		May have ill-defined, solid mass with irregular margins within breast
	Fever		
	May see retraction at site of previous abscess		May have a fairly well-circumscribed, rounded mass with posterior acoustic enhancement
	Differentiation between abscess and carcinoma based on clinical resolution		

BREAST

DISEASE PROCESS	CLINICAL, LABORATORY, AND RELATED FINDINGS	ETIOLOGY	ULTRASOUND FINDINGS
Cysts (single or multiple)	One of the most common masses in female breast (25% of masses)	Fibrocystic disease	Well-defined, smooth margin around echo-free interior; may be single or multiple
	Change in normal parenchymal breast pattern on mammogram	Localized fluid-filled ducts	Well-defined, thin walls
			Posterior acoustic enhancement
	Patient will experience pain correlated with palpation of nodules		Generally round or oval
	May change with menstrual cycle		May have reverberation artifact beneath anterior wall
	Palpable or nonpalpable mass		Occasionally may appear to have septations when two cysts are located adjacent to one another

DISEASE PROCESS	CLINICAL, LABORATORY, AND RELATED FINDINGS	ETIOLOGY	ULTRASOUND FINDINGS
Ducts	Pregnancy	Ducts fill with colostrum and then milk (in lactating patients) or with cellular and fatty debris (in older patients)	Ducts become enlarged; stellated appearance with anechoic echo pattern
	Lactation postpartum		Internal diameter 6–8 mm
Galactocele	Pain	Localized accumulation of milk behind obstructed lactiferous duct	Appears as a mass with well-defined margins
	Lactation may cause enlarged, hard breast		Low-level, uniform echoes within
Hematoma	Pain	Usually related to trauma or can follow needle aspiration biopsy	May appear as a weakly echogenic region of architectural distortion with various levels of echogenicity
	Swelling or palpable mass	Can occur without trauma in patients with blood disorder	Appearance changes according to stage of reorganization

HEMATOMA

BREAST

DISEASE PROCESS	CLINICAL, LABORATORY, AND RELATED FINDINGS	ETIOLOGY	ULTRASOUND FINDINGS
Solid masses			
Benign	Palpable breast thickening, hardening, and lumpiness; nontender	Fibroadenoma in majority of cases	Usually solitary
			Solid homogeneous mass
	Most common benign mass in females 15–35 yrs of age is fibroadenoma	Occurs from proliferation of connective and epithelial tissues	Round or oval lesions measuring a few mm to 8 cm
			Smoothly marginated, well-circumscribed mass
			May be lobulated
			Moderate internal echoes
			Variable levels of acoustic attenuation
Malignant	Evidence of mass and microcalcifications on mammogram	Most common malignant mass is infiltrating ductal carcinoma	Solid mass, hypoechoic
		Medullary carcinoma	Variably shaped with irregular contour

DISEASE PROCESS	CLINICAL, LABORATORY, AND RELATED FINDINGS	ETIOLOGY	ULTRASOUND FINDINGS
	If palpable, mass is usually hard, fixed, and painless	Infiltrating lobular carcinoma	Contains weak internal echoes
	Patient may note skin changes	Mucirous carcinoma	Variation of normal parenchymal echo distribution
	Receding nipple (advanced cases)	Tubular carcinoma	Majority have mild to significant acoustic attenuation
	Discharge (advanced cases)	Papillary carcinoma	

SOLID MASSES

CHEST

DISEASE PROCESS	CLINICAL, LABORATORY, AND RELATED FINDINGS	ETIOLOGY	ULTRASOUND FINDINGS
Atelectasis	Shortness of breath	Causes may include:	In association with pleural effusion, appears as a solid structure projecting into and out of the pleural fluid during respiration
	Pneumothorax prevents visualization of pleural space	• Trauma	
		• Emphysema	
		• Pneumonia	
		• Neoplasms	If collapse is partial, may see highly reflective alveoli with reverberation artifacts and acoustic shadowing
Pleural effusion	Variable dyspnea	Transudate	Echo-free space with well-defined borders, roughly triangular in shape, seen above the hemidiaphragm, bounded by the lung superiorly (parietal pleura) and the diaphragm inferiorly
	Bulging of intercostal spaces (large effusion)	Organization of inflammatory exudate	
	Diminished and delayed chest movement on involved side		

DISEASE PROCESS	CLINICAL, LABORATORY, AND RELATED FINDINGS	ETIOLOGY	ULTRASOUND FINDINGS
	Hemi- or bilateral opacification on chest radiograph; may be associated with loss of lung volume		Seen best in longitudinal plane
			In transverse plane, appears as a crescent-shaped fluid collection (anechoic) lateral, posterior, and superior to spleen or liver surface
			Able to differentiate solid from complex cystic involvement of pleural space, parenchyma, and surrounding soft tissue
			As intrapulmonary process becomes more aggressive, less well-defined borders and possibly irregular septa are seen

PLEURAL EFFUSION

FLUID
COLLECTIONS

FLUID COLLECTIONS

DISEASE PROCESS	CLINICAL, LABORATORY, AND RELATED FINDINGS	ETIOLOGY	ULTRASOUND FINDINGS
Fluid collections	Pain may or may not be present	Usually seromatous inflammatory process	Variably shaped, anechoic fluid collection that changes when patient changes position; with complications becomes more complex; may see septa
	Bulging or bloating of skin surface due to fluid collection arising in or involving subcutaneous plane, musculofascial plane, peritoneal surface, or intra-abdominal compartments	Abscess	Within peritoneal cavity, fluid collections conform to cavity contour
		Malignant process	
		Trauma with resultant loculated hematoma, lymphocele, or urinoma	Retroperitoneal fluid is usually lentiform or elliptically shaped, displacing kidneys or psoas muscles
			Posterior acoustic enhancement occurs with hematomas and serous fluid, but to a lesser degree with abscesses

DISEASE PROCESS	CLINICAL, LABORATORY, AND RELATED FINDINGS	ETIOLOGY	ULTRASOUND FINDINGS
Abscess	Pain	Surgery	Appears as complex mass with debris
	Fever	Trauma	Irregular borders; may appear thick-walled; may appear septated
	↑ WBC	Bowel perforation	May have acoustic shadowing if contains air
	Most aggressive process displacing adjacent organs		Difficult to distinguish from hematoma
Ascites	When free fluid levels increase, patient experiences fluctuant, painless swelling of abdomen	Exudative due to inflammation (e.g., neoplasm, infection)	Free-moving, anechoic fluid collection
	Hypoalbuminemia	Transudative due to obstruction of venous return (e.g., heart failure, nephrosis, cirrhosis)	Changes as patient changes position, moving to most dependent portion of body ▶

ASCITES

105

FLUID COLLECTIONS

DISEASE PROCESS	CLINICAL, LABORATORY, AND RELATED FINDINGS	ETIOLOGY	ULTRASOUND FINDINGS
Ascites (CONTINUED)			First seen in paracolic gutters, posterior cul-de-sac, and subhepatic space
			Bowel projects into fluid within inframesocolic space
Hematoma	Pain	Surgery	Depending on age of bleeding process, may appear echogenic (acute or chronic), complex (clotted with liquefaction), or anechoic (serous fluid remaining)
	↓ hematocrit (if hemorrhage continues or is large enough)	Trauma	
		Leaking aortic aneurysm	
		Bleeding neoplasm	
		Bleeding disorder	May see distortion of adjacent organs or displacement of vena cava or aorta
		Vasculitis	

DISEASE PROCESS	CLINICAL, LABORATORY, AND RELATED FINDINGS	ETIOLOGY	ULTRASOUND FINDINGS
			May appear to be well localized or a poorly defined infiltrative process
			Rectus sheath hematomas conform to the muscle while still causing bulging of its contour; muscle may appear asymmetric
Lymphocele	May be asymptomatic or may produce some abdominal discomfort or regionally referred pain	Extravasation of lymph into retroperitoneum

Trauma

Surgery resulting in damage to lymphatic channels (e.g., renal transplant) | Anechoic, walled-off fluid collection with posterior acoustic enhancement

May have irregular borders

May contain septa

May contain debris ▶ |

LYMPHOCELE

FLUID COLLECTIONS

DISEASE PROCESS	CLINICAL, LABORATORY, AND RELATED FINDINGS	ETIOLOGY	ULTRASOUND FINDINGS
Lymphocele *(CONTINUED)*			May be located in perinephric space; seen best in decubitus position, coronal view
Urinoma	Urine output may be normal or decreased due to extravasation	Trauma	Anechoic, walled-off fluid collection with posterior acoustic enhancement
		Surgery (e.g., renal transplant)	
	May be asymptomatic or may produce some abdominal discomfort	Subacute or chronic urinary obstruction resulting in perforation of the collecting system	May have irregular borders
			May contain septa
			May compress adjacent tissue
	Palpable flank mass		Usually located in perinephric space; seen best in decubitus position, coronal view
			May be seen within cul-de-sac

NECK MASSES

NECK MASSES

DISEASE PROCESS	CLINICAL, LABORATORY, AND RELATED FINDINGS	ETIOLOGY	ULTRASOUND FINDINGS
Branchial cleft cyst	Majority of patients are children	Persistence of embryonic branchial cleft remnant	Solitary unilateral mass separate from thyroid gland
	Patient presents with lateral neck mass, appearing at angle of mandible		Predominantly cystic, with posterior acoustic enhancement
	Usually anterior to the common carotid artery, along anterior border of the sternocleidomastoid muscle		May contain low-level dependent echoes
	Rx is exploration and resection		Cannot be differentiated sonographically from abscess
Lymphadenopathy	Palpable mass in region of node enlargement	Result of metastatic head or neck carcinomas, inflammation, or lymphoma	Enlarged nodular lesions of variable size
	May be unilateral or bilateral		Can see single enlarged node or, if multiple, appears as bulky, hypoechoic mass that may envelop or displace adjacent vasculature
	Other clinical findings dependent on etiology		

DISEASE PROCESS	CLINICAL, LABORATORY, AND RELATED FINDINGS	ETIOLOGY	ULTRASOUND FINDINGS
			Usually homogeneous
			May appear complex, primarily cystic
			Poor posterior acoustic enhancement
			Color Doppler demonstrating flow will distinguish vascular structures from lymphadenopathy
			Check for hepatomegaly, ascites, hydronephrosis, splenomegaly

LYMPHADENOPATHY

NEUROSONOLOGY

DISEASE PROCESS	CLINICAL, LABORATORY, AND RELATED FINDINGS	ETIOLOGY	ULTRASOUND FINDINGS
Agenesis of corpus callosum	Clinical significance uncertain; associated CNS anomalies common • Dandy–Walker malformation • NTD's • Microcephaly • Pyramidal tract abnormalities	Variable • Genetic factors (20%) • Vascular lesion or inflammation of commissural formation before 12 wks (complete) • Destruction of previously well-formed corpus callosum after 12 wks (partial) • Metabolic abnormalities	Marked separation of dilated frontal horns and bodies of lateral ventricles May have absent CSP Sharply angled superior-lateral peaks of lateral ventricles Third ventricle dilatation and elevation Cerebral sulci radiate vertically away from third ventricle Pericallosal artery loop lost on color 80% have associated anomalies

DISEASE PROCESS	CLINICAL, LABORATORY, AND RELATED FINDINGS	ETIOLOGY	ULTRASOUND FINDINGS
Arteriovenous malformation			
(See under Fetal cranial, spinal, and CNS abnormalities, p. 161)			
Dandy-Walker malformation			
(See under Fetal cranial, spinal, and CNS abnormalities, p. 163)			
Germinal matrix hemorrhage (progressing)	Most common type of bleed among premature infants	Fragile subependymal germinal matrix capillary ruptures, most typically at the junction of the caudothalamic groove ▶	(See progressive grading scale below)
	Most will be seen by the 7th day of life, although generally occur during the first 24–28 hrs		

GERMINAL MATRIX HEMORRHAGE (PROGRESSING)

DISEASE PROCESS	CLINICAL, LABORATORY, AND RELATED FINDINGS	ETIOLOGY	ULTRASOUND FINDINGS
Germinal matrix hemorrhage (progressing) *(CONTINUED)*		Effects of prematurity and birth asphyxia, myocardial failure, or pneumothorax	
		Grading system (below) assumes that bleed began in subependymal region; bleeding of parenchyma, thalami, basal ganglia, or choroid plexus are different processes	
Grade 0	Baseline normal scan		Normal exam with no evidence of hemorrhage
Grade 1 Subependymal hemorrhage (SEH)	Sudden drop in hematocrit and PO_2 Presence of blood in CSF	Blood confined to germinal matrix	Highly echogenic lesion at the caudothalamic groove, located at the head of the caudate nucleus; is adjacent to and inferior and lateral to the lateral ventricle on coronal view

DISEASE PROCESS	CLINICAL, LABORATORY, AND RELATED FINDINGS	ETIOLOGY	ULTRASOUND FINDINGS
	Patient has good potential for normal neurologic development if confined to Grade I		Ranges from 2 mm to 1 cm in size
	Majority of cases resolve completely, with no major evidence of specific neurologic deficits		With larger bleeds, focal ventricular compression may be seen
			On serial scans, bleed may: • Resolve, leaving a normal exam (majority of cases) • Resolve, leaving a subependymal cyst • Progress to intraventricular hemorrhage
Grade 2 Intraventricular hemorrhage (IVH without dilatation)	See Grade 1	SEH breaks through ventricle floor and bleeds through to ventricle	

GERMINAL MATRIX HEMORRHAGE (PROGRESSING)

DISEASE PROCESS	CLINICAL, LABORATORY, AND RELATED FINDINGS	ETIOLOGY	ULTRASOUND FINDINGS
Germinal matrix hemorrhage (progressing), *Grade 2 Intraventricular hemorrhage (IVH without dilatation) (CONTINUED)*			If seen early enough, small IVH may be visualized as fluid-echogenic blood layered in dependent portion of occipital horn
			Later, areas of bleed appear less well defined
			Prominent third and fourth ventricles
			Serial exams may demonstrate: • Return to normal size without intervention • Progression of IVH to include dilated ventricles

DISEASE PROCESS	CLINICAL, LABORATORY, AND RELATED FINDINGS	ETIOLOGY	ULTRASOUND FINDINGS
Grade 3 Intraventricular hemorrhage (IVH with dilatation)	Majority of cases result in some ventricular dilatation; treated with drug therapy, serial lumbar punctures, ventriculoperitoneal shunting	Expansion of ventricles by large amounts of blood (majority of cases)	Same as Grade 2, but with various degrees of ventriculomegaly
	Patient may have some mental retardation and motor problems	Patient: may have aqueductal obstruction resulting from clot or ventriculitis	Consistency and echogenicity change over time (see Grade 4)
	Posthemorrhagic hydrocephalus is the only type of hydrocephalus that may return to normal ventricular size		Serial exams may demonstrate: • Return to normal size without intervention • Stable, mild hydrocephalus • Progression to IPH
Grade 4 Intraparenchymal hemorrhage (IPH) [periventricular hemorrhage]	59% mortality rate ▶	Expansion of hemorrhage into brain parenchyma, usually the frontoparietal periventricular region of the cerebral hemisphere ▶	Hematoma extension lateral to the edge of the lateral ventricle(s) into the cerebral hemisphere ▶

GERMINAL MATRIX HEMORRHAGE (PROGRESSING)

119

NEUROSONOLOGY

DISEASE PROCESS	CLINICAL, LABORATORY, AND RELATED FINDINGS	ETIOLOGY	ULTRASOUND FINDINGS
Germinal matrix hemorrhage (progressing), *Grade 4 Intraparenchymal hemorrhage (CONTINUED)*	Survivors have ↑↑ incidence of major handicaps, including motor disabilities (86%) and cognitive defects (64%) such as spastic hemiparesis or asymmetric quadriparesis	Results in porencephaly due to necrosis and phagocytosis	May see extension into thalami or posterior fossa with marked asymmetry May see midline shift Four stages of resolving bleed into the cerebral parenchyma: • Stage 1: Hematoma is highly echogenic and homogeneous, with irregular margins • Stage 2: Center of hematoma appears hypoechoic to anechoic (due to beginning of clot resorption process), surrounded by echogenic rim; appears 1–2 weeks after bleed

DISEASE PROCESS	CLINICAL, LABORATORY, AND RELATED FINDINGS	ETIOLOGY	ULTRASOUND FINDINGS
			• Stage 3: Edge of well-demarcated hemorrhage becomes clearer as clot retracts to dependent portion of lesion with enlargement of ventricles; occurs 2–4 weeks after bleed
			• Stage 4: Hematoma appears anechoic due to complete necrosis of area; porencephalic cyst left, directly proportional to size of original lesion; occurs 2–3 months after bleed
			Periventricular infarction remains

GERMINAL MATRIX HEMORRHAGE (PROGRESSING)

DISEASE PROCESS	CLINICAL, LABORATORY, AND RELATED FINDINGS	ETIOLOGY	ULTRASOUND FINDINGS
Holoprosencephaly (See under Fetal cranial, spinal, and CNS abnormalities, p. 164)			
Hydranencephaly (See under Fetal cranial, spinal, and CNS abnormalities, p. 166)			
Hydrocephalus	Occurs from 0.5–3.0 times per 1,000 live births with varying degrees of neurologic impairment	A progressive ↑ in volume of ventricles 2° to a relative obstruction of CSF under pressure; may be partial or complete obstruction	Ventriculomegaly as evidenced by atria measuring >10 mm
	↑ Head size with continuing ↑ in circumference		Depending on etiology, can be unilateral or bilateral
	Increased intracranial pressure	Secondary to: Aqueductal stenosis	Choroid plexus, thickness appears relatively decreased as ventriculomegaly increases

DISEASE PROCESS	CLINICAL, LABORATORY, AND RELATED FINDINGS	ETIOLOGY	ULTRASOUND FINDINGS
	Headache	Hemorrhage	Posterior horn decreases first; Anterior horn increases last
	Vomiting	Infection	
	Variable reduction in the level of consciousness	Intracranial mass	>70% have associated anomalies of CNS, renal and cardiac origin
		In association with other anomalies:	
		• Dandy Walker malformation	
		• Arnold-Chiari malformation	
		• Arachnoid cysts	
		• AV malformation	
Intracerebral hemorrhage	Variable symptoms consisting of signs of increased intracranial pressure, including:	Hemorrhage due to trauma, birth trauma, blood dyscrasia (leukemia, thrombocytopenia, hemophilia, etc.)	Assymetric, echogenic mass usually seen in frontal or parietal lobe or, rarely, in cerebrum or brain stem
	• Bulging anterior fontanelle	▶	May be small or (rarely) massive
	• Lethargy		▶
	• Irritability		
	▶		

INTRACEREBRAL HEMORRHAGE

123

DISEASE PROCESS	CLINICAL, LABORATORY, AND RELATED FINDINGS	ETIOLOGY	ULTRASOUND FINDINGS
Intracerebral hemorrhage *(CONTINUED)*	• Hemiparesis • Hydrocephalus • Convulsions Bloody spinal tap	Usually found in association with subdural or extradural hemorrhage	Midline structures and ventricles are displaced by mass that appears as acute hemorrhage and undergoes the various reabsorption stages May see variable degrees of hydrocephalus Slow resolution eventually leaves area of anechoic porencephaly on follow-up exam; does not exhibit Doppler signal within lesion
Intracranial hemorrhage (ICH)	Most common and most serious cause of low birth weight or preterm newborn morbidity and mortality	(All-inclusive term for any hemorrhagic process, specifically those listed below)	General findings include: • Initially high echogenicity without acoustic shadowing

DISEASE PROCESS	CLINICAL, LABORATORY, AND RELATED FINDINGS	ETIOLOGY	ULTRASOUND FINDINGS
	2:1 male:female ratio	Prematurity; germinal matrix bleed associated with gestation of less than 34 weeks and/or birth weight less than 1500 g; 25–40% incidence	• Slightly decreasing echogenicity over the next week
	May include:		• At 1–2 weeks: moderately echogenic rim surrounding central sonolucency as clot beings to dissolve
	• Seizures	Congenital anomalies	
	• Enlarged head size	Genetic syndromes	
	• Bulging fontanelle	Trauma at delivery	• After 2 weeks: anechoic area between echogenic rim surrounding anechoic center gradually shrinks
	• Change in muscular tone and activity	Apnea resulting in:	
	• Vascular hypotension	• Anoxia/hypoxia	
	• Cyanosis or pallor	• Asphyxia	• Porencephalic cysts form as hematoma retracts
	• Respiratory distress	• Increased blood pressure	
	• Poor sucking and feeding		▶
	Decreased hematocrit	Other precipitous increases in intracranial blood pressure due to:	
	Presence of blood in CSF		
		▶	

125

INTRACRANIAL HEMORRHAGE (ICH)

DISEASE PROCESS	CLINICAL, LABORATORY, AND RELATED FINDINGS	ETIOLOGY	ULTRASOUND FINDINGS
Intracranial hemorrhage (ICH) *(CONTINUED)*		• Infant on respirator • Suctioning of infant • IRDS • Coagulation disorders • Patent ductus arteriosus	Fluctuating pattern of cerebral blood flow velocities and fluctuating RI may indicate increased risk of ICH
Neural tube defects (See under Fetal cranial, spinal, and CNS abnormalities, pp. 160–172)			
Papilloma of choroid plexuses	Occurs in children <2 yrs of age Rapidly increasing head size due to hydrocephalus	Usually benign; epithelial tumor of the choroid plexus; ↑ secretion of CSF or obstruction of CSF flow; more common in the lateral ventricles in children Rare	Large, echogenic mass within the dilated ventricle; echogenicity similar to that of normal choroid May compress adjacent structures Usually unilateral

DISEASE PROCESS	CLINICAL, LABORATORY, AND RELATED FINDINGS	ETIOLOGY	ULTRASOUND FINDINGS
Periventricular leukomalacia	Not a common cerebral insult; occurs primarily in mature neonatal population; when occurring in premature population, contributes to neurologic deficits	CNS dysfunction due to hypoxic ischemic insult, infection, or embolism sustained during the perinatal period; results in diffuse cerebral edema, infarction, and focal necrosis of watershed zones between anterior and middle and middle and posterior cerebral arteries	May initially see nothing
			May see bilateral hyperechoic margins of lateral ventricles and adjacent to region of foramen of Monro
	Infant often pale and limp at birth	Can result from:	Increased linear echogenic pattern can be focal, representing arterial distribution alterations, or extend into cerebrum, representing venous infarctions
	Seizures may occur during resuscitation or later	• Maternal hypotension	
	Hypotonia and hyporeflexia may occur, especially in lower extremities	• Umbilical cord compression	Important to image using perpendicular angle of transducer to region; should be resolved as discrete linear structures
	Marked retinal hemorrhages often occur	• Uteroplacental insufficiency	
	▶	▶	▶

PERIVENTRICULAR LEUKOMALACIA

127

NEUROSONOLOGY

DISEASE PROCESS	CLINICAL, LABORATORY, AND RELATED FINDINGS	ETIOLOGY	ULTRASOUND FINDINGS
Periventricular leukomalacia *(CONTINUED)*	Prognosis depends on infant's size and severity of asphytic attack, but generally is poor	• Noncentral nervous system problems such as meconium aspiration, cardiac abnormalities, or hyaline membrane disease	Usually appears bilaterally and symmetrically
	Results in severe neurologic deficits, including:		May be less echogenic than or as highly echogenic as acute hemorrhage
	• Spastic diplegia or dysplegia (almost every case)		Remainder of brain has normal echogenic appearance
	• Visual defects		
	• Marked intellectual developmental delay occurs often		To confirm diagnosis, cystic lesions indicating liquefaction are seen on serial exams 1–4 wks later, most frequently at the posterior striations above the lateral ventricular trigones
			Infrequently, concomitant intraventricular enlargement or hemorrhages may occur

DISEASE PROCESS	CLINICAL, LABORATORY, AND RELATED FINDINGS	ETIOLOGY	ULTRASOUND FINDINGS
Subdural hematoma	Occurs more commonly in: • Large infants delivered by primagravid women • Infants born by breech delivery • Infants delivered precipitously by multiparous women Manifested by: • Pallor, cyanosis, and high-pitched cry appearing shortly after birth • Frequent seizures • Hypotonia • Hemiparesis (possibly) • Presence of retinal hemorrhages • Bloody subdural tap ▶	Uncommon; incidence ranges from 3–18% Venous in origin; initiated by dural venous lacerations or rupture of the unsupported bridging veins over the convexities between the brain and dural sinuses Usually associated with trauma, or, less commonly, with birth or postoperative trauma	Difficult to visualize unless >2 cm Variable size May be unilateral or bilateral Seen as anechoic spaces separating bony calvarium from brain parenchyma Gryi and sulci are well demonstrated due to compression by fluid Midline shift is 2° sign (especially if hematoma is unilateral) ▶

DISEASE PROCESS	CLINICAL, LABORATORY, AND RELATED FINDINGS	ETIOLOGY	ULTRASOUND FINDINGS
Subdural hematoma *(CONTINUED)*	• Tense or bulging fontanelle CT and MRI are modalities of choice for diagnosis		Widening of intrahemispheric fissure or tentorium (depending on site of origin) may be only ultrasound finding
TORCH group (antenatally acquired infections)	Diagnosis usually made in neonatal period Maternal symptoms are uncommon	Toxoplasmosis Other (e.g., syphilis, hepatitis) Rubella Cytomegalovirus (CMV) Herpes simplex virus	↑ Echogenicity in affected region likely due to basophilic deposits in arterial walls or hypercellular arterial walls
Toxoplasmosis	The second most common infection in the world Clinically, resembles other TORCH entities Infant may be asymptomatic, but this depends on when infection is acquired	Protozoal Parasitic infection	Hepatosplenomegaly May see hydrocephalus Intracranial calcifications are visualized throughout the brain, without specific distribution

DISEASE PROCESS	CLINICAL, LABORATORY, AND RELATED FINDINGS	ETIOLOGY	ULTRASOUND FINDINGS
	Prognosis related to severity of neuropathology Infant may present with congenital septic indications, such as: • Jaundice • Hepatosplenomegaly • Purpura • Anemia • CNS involvement • Chorioretinitis • Thrombocytopenia • Microcephaly	Congenital infection following maternal infection during pregnancy; affects fetus variably, depending on the trimester in which mother was infected The later the exposure, the higher the risk of fetal transmission; the earlier the exposure, the greater the severity of infection	Microcephaly ↑ placental thickness
Rubella	Presents similarly to other TORCH entities ▶		

TORCH GROUP

NEUROSONOLOGY

DISEASE PROCESS	CLINICAL, LABORATORY, AND RELATED FINDINGS	ETIOLOGY	ULTRASOUND FINDINGS
TORCH group, *Rubella* (*CONTINUED*)	May present with congenital malformations such as microcephaly and cardiac disease (includes 15–20% of those born to mothers who had it) Definitive diagnosis based on virologic or serologic confirmation	Maternal viral infection early in pregnancy (first 12 wks) leads to infection of the placenta, which seeds virus to fetus Rare since widespread vaccine availability	Usually microcephaly with calcification occurring infrequently (although massive calcification has been reported) May see small, multiple, subependymal cysts May see echogenic foci at basal ganglia
Cytomegalovirus (CMV)	The most common CNS infection in neonates (1–2% most populations)	DNA-containing virus classified as a herpes virus with its own genus Maternal primary infection during pregnancy results in infection of fetus through placenta	Presence of punctate intracranial periventricular calcifications, most typically scattered along ventricular wall and at the thalamus and basal ganglia (representing arterial vasculature); may or may not shadow

DISEASE PROCESS	CLINICAL, LABORATORY, AND RELATED FINDINGS	ETIOLOGY	ULTRASOUND FINDINGS
	98% of infants exposed are asymptomatic, but when symptomatic, infants are quite ill	Congenital infection has been reported in consecutive pregnancies, with no symptoms in subsequent infants	May see ventriculomegaly with echogenic walls
	Clinical manifestations include:	Infant may also acquire virus through contact with infected cervix in delivery or through ingestion of virus in breast milk	May see small, multiple subependymal cysts (presumably due to neural cell necrosis)
	• Hepatosplenomegaly		
	• Hyperbilirubinemia		May see prominent cisterna magna
	• Thrombocytopenia with purpura or petechiae		Hepatomegaly
	• Gestational prematurity		May see ascites
	• IUGR		Delayed studies will show persistent visualization of above findings
	• Encephalitis		
	• Microcephaly		
	Definitive diagnosis based on virologic or serologic confirmation		

TORCH GROUP

133

NEUROSONOLOGY

DISEASE PROCESS	CLINICAL, LABORATORY, AND RELATED FINDINGS	ETIOLOGY	ULTRASOUND FINDINGS
Torch group *(CONTINUED)*			
Herpes simplex	If acquired in utero, associated with: • Sepsis • Lethargy • Seizures • Herpetic lesions or vesicles (50% of cases) Presents in first to third week of life Diffuse encephalitis High mortality rate (50%) Sequelae include psychomotor retardation and ocular defects	Herpes simplex virus (type 2) Major source of transmission is through mother's infected cervix or lower genital tract at time of delivery May be acquired in utero through placental transmission or intact chorioamnion	Microcephaly May see intracranial periventricular calcifications May see ventriculomegaly Severe brain damage may result in compressed, thin cerebral mantle

OBSTETRICS - GYNECOLOGY

Normal uterine size
prepuberty: 1.0–3.3 cm
(length); 0.5–1.0 cm (width)
postpuberty (nulliparous):
7 × 4 × 4 cm (multiparous);
8.2 × 6.2 × 6.2 cm
postmenopause: 3.5–6.5 cm
(length); 1.2–1.8 cm (AP);
2 cm (width)

Normal ovarian size
prepuberty: 15 × 2.5 × 3 mm

postpuberty: 30 × 20 × 15 mm
(normal vol 6.5 cm^3)
postmenopause: size
atrophied; significant when
one is 2 × vol of other or
>7.1 cm^3

Normal endometrial thickness
menses: 0–5 mm
proliferative phase: 5–7 mm
secretory phase: 7–12 mm

postmenopause HRT: <8 mm
postmenopause non-HRT:
(without bleeding) 3.2 mm

Doppler flow patterns
resting ovary: low velocity,
high-impedance waveform
ovulatory ovary: high-velocity,
low-impedance, declining
before ovulation, then
rising after ovulation
uterus: normal RI mean 0.84

MENSTRUAL AGE* ULTRASOUND FINDINGS[†]

OBSTETRICS

The pregnant uterus

	Identification of gestational sac may occur when serum β-hCG is 200 IU/L
3½–4 wks	Decidual reaction endometrium; endovaginally, gestational sac measures 2–3 mm
5–6 wks	Transabdominally, gestational sac measures 1 cm; EHM visualized endovaginally
6–7 wks	Embryonic pole is seen adjacent to secondary yolk sac; pole measures 3–4 mm
7–8 wks	CRL (±5 days accuracy to 12 weeks gestation; ±3 days accuracy with 3–5 measurements)
	EM/EHM visualized transabdominally
8–10 wks	Developing placenta appears as thickened portion of gestational ring (decidua basalis), easily identified by 12 weeks; *Endovaginally:* can easily visualize amnion surrounding embryo as it approaches chorion

*Menstrual age is defined as the number of weeks since the first day of the last normal menstrual period (EGA, Estimated Gestational Age, used synonymously).

[†]Overall accuracy rate: 13–15 wks, ±7 days; 16–19 wks, ±7–10 days; 20–29 wks, ±14 days; 30–40 wks, ±21 days. (Normal variations in fetal size increase with menstrual age.)

MENSTRUAL AGE	ULTRASOUND FINDINGS
12 wks	BPD, FL, HC, and AC can be measured as separate parameters
	Bladder visualized; amnionchorion fused; three-vessel cord
13–20 wks	Most accurate BPD measurements (±1 wk)
	Most accurate FL measurement
	Stomach, bladder, and kidneys visualized routinely
18 wks	Bladder must be seen
The pregnant cervix	Examined translabially or endovaginally, measures 3–3.7 cm (range, 2–6 cm); in third trimester, noncervically effaced cervix; cerclage appears as bright, echogenic focus at external os
14–16 wks	Visualization of incompetent cervix considered if cervix measures less than 3 cm
	EV or translabially: Cervical measurement shortened and funneling seen past internal os.
	Transabdominally: As widening occurs, area of pointed sonolucency toward external os (funneling) seen

VIEW ULTRASOUND FINDINGS

Fetal cardiac evaluation (minimal)

Four-chamber

Fetal heart approximately 30% of thoracic size

Apex of heart to left (levocardiac)

Atria and ventricles are symmetric

Interventricular septum is intact

Tricuspid valve is slightly more apical than mitral valve

LVOT

Evaluate continuity of LV into ascending aortic root and make sure that IVS is intact

RVOT

Evaluate continuity of RV into main pulmonary artery

RVOT and LVOT approximately equal in size

PLACENTAL GRADE	ULTRASOUND FINDINGS
Placental grading scale	
Grade 0	Homogeneous echo pattern bounded by smoooth chorionic plate
	Grade 0 placenta is normal up to 31–33 wks
Grade I	Decreased homogeneous echo pattern begins to become slightly uneven and broken up by echogenic changes as macroscopic calcifications appear
	40% of all babies delivered have Grade I placentas; normal, 31–36 wks
Grade II	Basilar and intraplacental calcifications begin to appear as comma-like densities extending into placental substance
	40% of all babies delivered have Grade II placentas; normal, 36–38 wks
Grade III	Diffuse calcifications are visualized; indentations of reflective chorionic plate and basilar plate into intraplacental perivillous septa are seen
	10–15% of term placentas are Grade III
Doppler	Normal Doppler waveform demonstrates low resistance patterns; RI and S/D ratios are lower in the ipsilateral site of placental implantation in first half of pregnancy

MENSTRUAL AGE   **ULTRASOUND FINDINGS**

Normal placenta

12 wks	Placenta visible; echogenic compared to myometrium; location easily seen
	Diffusely homogeneous
16 wks	Placenta is approximately the same size as the fetus; has reached its maximum final thickness (2–4 cm)
Over 16 wks	Placental calcifications increase exponentially beginning at about 29 wks
	50% of all placentas show some degree of calcification by 33 wks
	No additional calcification is seen in postmature placentas

ULTRASOUND FINDINGS	ETIOLOGY
Abnormal placental development	Some considerations:
Edematous (thick) placenta (> 5 cm)	Gestational diabetes
	Rh sensitization (erythroblastosis)
	Maternal infections (i.e., CMV, syphilis)
	Maternal congestive heart failure
	Molar pregnancy
	Twin-to-twin transfusion syndrome
	Chorioangioma
Thin placenta (< 1.5 cm,	Preeclampsia
	Essential hypertension
	IUGR
	Juvenile diabetes

OBSTETRICS-GYNECOLOGY

DISEASE PROCESS	CLINICAL, LABORATORY, AND RELATED FINDINGS	ETIOLOGY	ULTRASOUND FINDINGS
Placenta and amniotic fluid			
Abruptio placentae	Patient may have: • Vaginal bleeding • Hypovolemic shock • Rigid abdomen with pain • No symptoms Clinical findings will predominate; are usually proportional to degree of separation May result in fetal death	Insult to placental lining due to trauma, labor, maternal HTN, cocaine abuse, or idiopathic causes, resulting in premature separation or complete detachment Most separations are spontaneous and nontraumatic	Anechoic or complex collection beneath the placenta Sometimes appears thickened as clots form between myometrium and placenta, increasing placental thickness Hematoma may evolve to a complex pattern Blood may appear as fluid collection between chorion and amnion May be difficult to differentiate from intraplacental lesions or less severe retroplacental hemorrhage

DISEASE PROCESS	CLINICAL, LABORATORY, AND RELATED FINDINGS	ETIOLOGY	ULTRASOUND FINDINGS
Chorioangioma	Occurs in 1% of pregnancies	Benign vascular malformation of nontrophoblastic tumor	Enlarged placenta with variably sized tumors
	Larger lesions associated with:	Tumor may act as an arteriovenous shunt if large enough	Larger solitary lesion appears as well-circumscribed intraplacental mass which may demonstrate intratumoral color flow
	• Low birth weight		
	• Premature labor		Variable echo pattern from isoechoic to complex as related to placenta
	• Fetal death		
	• Fetal hydrops		May see fetal hydrops, cardiomegaly
	• Cardiomegaly		
	• CHF		Distinguished by normal echogenicity of placenta, ruling out hydatidiform mole's vesicular appearance

DISEASE PROCESS	CLINICAL, LABORATORY, AND RELATED FINDINGS	ETIOLOGY	ULTRASOUND FINDINGS
Placenta and amniotic fluid *(CONTINUED)*			
Infarct (placental)	Occurs with increasing frequency in preeclampsia and essential hypertension	Coagulative necrosis of villi due to progressive ureteroplacental circulation changes in pregnancy	Anechoic space at the maternal surface of the placenta with no color flow
	Most occur without significant complications, but depends on extent of infarct and on underlying cause	Changes associated with aging of the trophoblast, as indicated by fibrinoid degeneration, calcification, and ischemic infarction	Variable size Size of infarcts ranges from millimeters to 2–3 cm
Intervillous thrombosis	Most occur without significant complications	Intraplacental hemorrhage of RBC from fetus to intervillous space	Hypoechoic to anechoic lesion within the placenta with no color flow
	Occurs most commonly at placental base	Microscopically, consists of layers of laminated fibrin	Variable size, ranging from a few millimeters to several centimeters; round to oval shape

DISEASE PROCESS	CLINICAL, LABORATORY, AND RELATED FINDINGS	ETIOLOGY	ULTRASOUND FINDINGS
	Occurs in up to 50% of term placentas		Partial: portion of placenta overlies cervical os, but bulk is either anterior or posterior to area of os
	Occurs with increasing frequency in cases of Rh isoimmunization		Low-lying or marginal: placenta near the cervical os but not covering it
	Associated with complications at delivery and increased perinatal mortality		Posterior previa not likely if the distance between the head and the sacrum is less than 2 cm
Oligohydramnios	Maternal size small for dates	Reduction in amniotic fluid due to:	Largest pocket of amniotic fluid is less than 2 cm in its greatest axis; four-quadrant AFI, oligo
	If persistent, leads to hypoplastic lungs	• IUCR restriction	>8 cm
	Fetal compromise is highly likely	• Bilateral renal disease	▶
		• PROM	
		• Postmaturity	
		• Fetal death	

OBSTETRICS-GYNECOLOGY

DISEASE PROCESS	CLINICAL, LABORATORY, AND RELATED FINDINGS	ETIOLOGY	ULTRASOUND FINDINGS
Placenta and amniotic fluid, *Oligohydramnios* *(CONTINUED)*			When fluid volume plus mature placenta before 36 weeks presents, likelihood of IUGR increases Filling and emptying of fetal bladder rules out renal disease
Polyhydramnios	Maternal size large for dates May create clinical problems related to burden for mother, such as: • Discomfort; SOB • Premature labor • Premature separation of placenta • Prolapsed cord • Postpartum uterine atony	Increased amniotic fluid due to fluid secretions and resorption alterations of fetus or mother • Idiopathic cause (60% of cases) *Fetal origin (20%)* • Neural tube defect and/or other CNS defects • GI abnormalities such as TE fistula, esophageal and duodenal atresia	Excessive amniotic fluid surrounding fetus Fetal extremities seem to float away from body trunk Utilizing four-quadrant AFI, volume >20 cm After discovering increase in fluid amount, thorough exam of fetus may reveal: • Normal fetus

DISEASE PROCESS	CLINICAL, LABORATORY, AND RELATED FINDINGS	ETIOLOGY	ULTRASOUND FINDINGS
	Associated with fetal anomalies, such as: • Miscellaneous limb shortening conditions • CHF	• Ventral wall defects *Maternal origin (20%)* • Diabetes mellitus • Rh incompatibility • Multiple pregnancy	• Neural tube defect and associated findings • GI defect • Multiple gestation • Skeletal dysplasia • Congenital heart defects
Previa (placenta)	Occurs in 1:250 live births Painless maternal bleeding caused by separation of the placenta as lower uterine segment lengthens during late pregnancy	Lower uterine placental implantation covering the cervical os to some degree (from partial to complete obstruction) More common in patients with history of low C-section or myomectomy	Easily seen endovaginally Full bladder required for transabdominal approach Complete; bulk of placenta completely overlies the cervical os
Subchorionic fibrin deposition	No clinical significance	Laminated subchorionic fibrin	Anechoic or hypoechoic fluid collection beneath chorion; no color flow

OBSTETRICS-GYNECOLOGY

DISEASE PROCESS	CLINICAL, LABORATORY, AND RELATED FINDINGS	ETIOLOGY	ULTRASOUND FINDINGS
Abortion			
General information	Vaginal bleeding before 20th week, with subsequent pregnancy loss; occurs in 15% of all pregnancies	Disruption of endometrial tissue due to: • Genetic defect of embryo • Hormone level not adequate to support pregnancy • External causes (e.g., viral infections, drugs, trauma)	May see hypoechoic area around gestational sac representing subchorionic hemorrhage Use prolate elipse formula to estimate volume: (length × width × height × .52) Those <¼ sac size or <60 ml usually go on to have normal pregnancy
Anembryonic gestation	Uterus exam will find size less than corresponding dates Patient will feel "less pregnant," with decrease in breast tenderness	Anembryonic gestation	Well-formed gestational sac No embryo parts seen within sac Gestation sac not appropriate for dates

DISEASE PROCESS	CLINICAL, LABORATORY, AND RELATED FINDINGS	ETIOLOGY	ULTRASOUND FINDINGS
	(+) β-hCG but not rising		*Transabdominally*
			Any sac >2.5 cm in diameter without internal embryonic/fetal echoes
			Endovaginally
			Any sac >1.6 cm without embryo; early pregnancy loss is likely
			May see fluid-fluid level within sac due to echogenic blood
			May see distortion in shape of sac
			Likely to see abnormal decidual reaction
Complete	Heavy vaginal bleeding	*See Abortion*	Normal endometrial canal; no evidence of IUP
	(+) but dropping hCG if recent event		▶

DISEASE PROCESS	CLINICAL, LABORATORY, AND RELATED FINDINGS	ETIOLOGY	ULTRASOUND FINDINGS
Abortion, *Complete* (*CONTINUED*)			Peritrophoblastic color flow low or absent
Embryonic demise	No tissue passed	Nonviable embryo retained in uterus	Embryo in gestational sac with no EHM; shifts when patient changes position
	Patient may or may not bleed		
	Dropping β-hCG level		May see retrochorionic hemorrhage
Incomplete	Some but not all products of conception expelled	*See Abortion*	Appearance varies and may include:
	Cervix dilated		• Irregular gestational sac
	(+) but dropping β-hCG		• Ill-defined embryo
			• Occasionally, clot or decidual tissue seen
			• May see dilated cervix
			• May see ↑ corpus luteal flow
			• Peritrophoblastic flow present

DISEASE PROCESS	CLINICAL, LABORATORY, AND RELATED FINDINGS	ETIOLOGY	ULTRASOUND FINDINGS
Threatened	25% have vaginal spotting or bleeding	Most commonly idiopathic	Complete gestational sac
	Cervix closed		Visible embryo with EHM (+++)
	(+) β-hCG		Crescent-shaped, anechoic ring within endometrial canal (may represent blood outside chorion or amnion)
	May or may not be accompanied by cramping pain		
	85–90% go on to normal delivery when EHM++		
Fetal abdominal abnormalities			
Ascites	Associated with:	Effusion of fluid into peritoneal cavity	May include visualization of:
	• Rh isoimmunization	▶	• Fetal abdominal ascites
	• Congenital heart anomalies		• Pleural effusion
	• Fetal anemia		• Pericardial effusion
	▶		▶

OBSTETRICS-GYNECOLOGY

DISEASE PROCESS	CLINICAL, LABORATORY, AND RELATED FINDINGS	ETIOLOGY	ULTRASOUND FINDINGS
Fetal abdominal abnormalities. *Ascites* (CONTINUED)	• Fetal tumors • In utero infections • GI-GU obstruction	Broad range of causes, all indicative of a poor prognosis for the fetus	• Hepatosplenomegaly • Cardiomegaly • Fetal peripheral edema (skin thickening) • Polyhydramnios • Scalp edema
Atresia			
DUODENAL	May or may not have increased AFP Associated with esophageal atresia, imperforate anus, small bowel and biliary atresia, cardiac anomalies 33% of cases associated with Down syndrome	Atresia resulting from incomplete recanalization of lumen or insufficient blood supply to bowel, usually at second part of duodenum, resulting in dilated, fluid-filled stomach and duodenal segment proximal to the atresia	Polyhydramnios "Double bubble"—abdomen visualized with nonperistaltic fluid between the two fluid structures; can connect two "bubbles" May visualize associated fetal heart abnormalities
ESOPHAGEAL	Associated with TE fistula	No known pattern	Polyhydramnios, often mild

DISEASE PROCESS	CLINICAL, LABORATORY, AND RELATED FINDINGS	ETIOLOGY	ULTRASOUND FINDINGS
	Increased AFP	Failure of esophageal endodermal proliferation	Persistent serial inability to demonstrate fluid in stomach
	Associated with cardiovascular and GU anomalies and imperforate anus	Blind end proximal esophagus	
Choledochal cyst	No other associated abnormalities seen in utero	Diverticulum of common bile duct, hepatic duct, or cystic duct	Appears as cystic mass within abdomen distinct from gallbladder
			May have "double bubble" sign, but the two areas do not connect
			Amniotic fluid normal
			Ultrasound differentials: • Duplication cyst • Mesenteric cyst • Ovarian cyst

OBSTETRICS-GYNECOLOGY

DISEASE PROCESS	CLINICAL, LABORATORY, AND RELATED FINDINGS	ETIOLOGY	ULTRASOUND FINDINGS
Fetal abdominal abnormalities *(CONTINUED)*			
Gastroschisis	Mom may be S > D Increased AFP Up to 50% have ↑ ACE Associated with: • Volvulus • Meckel's diverticulum	Defect of abdominal wall with herniation of abdominal viscera; occurs in 1:10,000 births Probably due to an embryonic vascular accident in which abnormal involution of right umbilical vein occurs at 6 wks gestational age	Discontinuity of anterior abdominal wall, out of which fluid-containing bowel protrudes freely into amniotic fluid; cord usually inserts at right of defect Polyhydramnios No covering membrane; abdominal contents float freely in amniotic fluid Extrophied gut appears intensely echogenic, thick, and increasingly dilated with time
Omphalocele	Increased AFP		

DISEASE PROCESS	CLINICAL, LABORATORY, AND RELATED FINDINGS	ETIOLOGY	ULTRASOUND FINDINGS
	Up to 50% have ↑ AFP	Defect of anterior abdominal wall occurs in 1:4000 births	Polyhydramnios (not always severe)
	Associated with a large number of congenital anomalies, including CV and GI anomalies; 40–60% have chromosomal anomalies	Fusion of lateral ectomeso-dermal folds fails; intestinal loops fail to return to abdominal cavity	Herniated mass can contain bowel only, or liver, spleen, bladder, uterus, tubes, stomach, or ovaries
	May be part of Beckwith-Weideman syndrome, cloacal extrophy, or pentalogy of Cantrell	Note: making a distinction between prenatal ruptured omphalocele and gastroschisis is not always possible, but it is not essential since both conditions require a pediatric surgeon to be present at birth	Umbilical cord inserts into base of herniated mass; typically has covering amnionic membrane
			May see findings associated with malformation syndromes
Teratoma	Elevated AFP and solid appearance suggest higher risk of malignancy ▶	Dysgenesis of three germ cell layers during cellular development ▶	Complex, primarily solid mass due to high vascularity and cellular composition ▶

DISEASE PROCESS	CLINICAL, LABORATORY, AND RELATED FINDINGS	ETIOLOGY	ULTRASOUND FINDINGS
Fetal abdominal abnormalities, *Teratoma* *(CONTINUED)*	Cystic appearance tends to be benign Relatively good prognosis	Usually occurs in sacral area, less often in cervical area, but may occur anywhere	Polyhydramnios May achieve large proportions May see hydrops fetalis May contain areas of calcifications with acoustic shadowing
Fetal cervicothoracic abnormalities			
Congenital diaphragmatic hernia	Occurs more frequently in males (2:1) >50% mortality rate Pulmonary hypoplasia Associated anomalies include CNS, CV, and GI anomalies	Defect in diaphragm, with resulting displacement of abdominal contents into thoracic cavity Usually unilateral, left-sided	Entire heart displaced to side opposite defect Polyhydramnios Degree of abdominal contents in thorax variable; stomach, bowel, spleen

DISEASE PROCESS	CLINICAL, LABORATORY, AND RELATED FINDINGS	ETIOLOGY	ULTRASOUND FINDINGS
Cystic adenomatoid malformation	*Macroscopic* Type I: Good prognosis Type II: Associated with GI-GU anomalies *Microscopic* Type III: Poor prognosis	Rare Cystic replacement of lung tissue, usually just one lobe of the lung	Can be unilobular, unilateral, or bilateral Compression of normal lung tissue; can create mediastinal shift Polyhydramnios Fetal hydrops; skin thickening Type I: Variably sized cyst >2 cm Type II: Cysts <1 cm Type III: Large noncystic lesions containing many microscopic cysts
Cystic hygroma	Elevated AFP is common but may be normal ▶		

DISEASE PROCESS	CLINICAL, LABORATORY, AND RELATED FINDINGS	ETIOLOGY	ULTRASOUND FINDINGS
Fetal cervicothoracic abnormalities, *Cystic hygroma* *(CONTINUED)*	Associated with: • Turner's syndrome • Omphalocele • Cardiac anomalies • Trisomies 13, 18, and 21	Defect of lymphatico-venous communication, usually associated with intradermoid lymphangiectasia, resulting in overdistention of jugular lymphatic sacs	Large fluid-filled mass arising from posterior, most often lateral, or anterior aspect of fetal neck (most common) or from the chest wall Mass has thin, wavy surrounding membrane Multiseptated Nonimmune fetal hydrops is common AFI may be low, normal, or increased Enlarged, edematous placenta is common

DISEASE PROCESS	CLINICAL, LABORATORY, AND RELATED FINDINGS	ETIOLOGY	ULTRASOUND FINDINGS
Ectopia cordis	Isolated finding Incompatible with life	Extremely rare Defect of anterior chest wall fusion results in ectopic placement of heart	Presence of heart, which demonstrates characteristic cardiac pulsations, anterior to ventral chest wall Color flow confirms extrathoracic FHM
Pericardial effusion	Associated with: • Fetal cardiac abnormalities • Rh factor abnormalities	CHF Idiopathic Related to isoimmune entities	Fetal heart surrounded by anechoic fluid >2 mm Fetal hydrops (pleural and peritoneal)
Pleural effusion	Associated with fetal hydrops, chromosomal anomalies	Causes are variable May be primary or associated with other disease processes, e.g., nonimmune or immune anemia Abnormal chromosomes	Polyhydramnios Cystic collections in one or both hemithorax Lungs within fluid appear as small, echogenic masses

OBSTETRICS-GYNECOLOGY

Fetal cranial, spinal, and CNS abnormalities

DISEASE PROCESS	CLINICAL, LABORATORY, AND RELATED FINDINGS	ETIOLOGY	ULTRASOUND FINDINGS
Anencephaly	Mother large for dates	Failure of neural tube to close at cephalic end	Polyhydramnios 50%, due to CSF dumping directly into sac
	↑ AFP and ACE	Occurs between second and third wks of development	↑↑ fetal activity
	Associated with spina bifida (17%)	No brain development above stem	Skull base visualized; none to small amounts of loose brain tissue present (cerebrovasculosis)
	Occurs in 1:1000 births	Fetal dysphagia is typical (contributes to ↑amniotic fluid levels)	No cranium visualized
	Open area of defect not covered by skin		Face and orbits easily visualized (lens in lower lateral orbit)

DISEASE PROCESS	CLINICAL, LABORATORY, AND RELATED FINDINGS	ETIOLOGY	ULTRASOUND FINDINGS
Arachnoid cyst	Contains clear CSF	Collection of CSF due to adhesions of meninges	Most cysts discovered during evaluation for other anomalies
		Fluid is usually trapped in areas of cisterns (in particular, areas of se la turcica, posterior to third ventricle, and posterior fossa)	Thin, anechoic mass; may be septated; seen between brain and dura, usually centrally
			May see hydrocephalus if cysts occur in certain areas
			Does not connect to ventricles; will not see color flow in mass
Arteriovenous malformation	Cardiac failure	Failure of embryonic arteriovenous shunts to be replaced by capillaries	May manifest as unusually shaped cystic lesions, such as vein of Galen aneurysm
	Doppler examinations provide confirmation		May present as discrete areas of increased echogenicity due to hemangiomas with color flow

▶

OBSTETRICS-GYNECOLOGY

DISEASE PROCESS	CLINICAL, LABORATORY, AND RELATED FINDINGS	ETIOLOGY	ULTRASOUND FINDINGS
Fetal cranial, spinal, and CNS abnormalities, *Arteriovenous malformation (CONTINUED)*			Vein of Galen aneurysm is easily confused with posterior fossa or porencephalic cysts
Arnold-Chiari II malformation	Direct postnatal findings in spectrum of dysraphic anomalies	Anterior and posterior neural tube closure defects	"Lemon" sign seen in second trimester
	↑ MSAFP	Associated with dysraphism of the spine and meningomyelocele, downward displacement of the fourth ventricle, posterior fossa structures into widened foramen magnum; cisterna magnum obliterated	Displacement of cerebellar tonsils into foramen magnum; cisterna magna obliterated; "Banana" sign
	↑ AFP		Ventriculomegaly; wide interhemispheric fissure
			Large massa intermedia fills third ventricle

DISEASE PROCESS	CLINICAL, LABORATORY, AND RELATED FINDINGS	ETIOLOGY	ULTRASOUND FINDINGS
			Low, flattened tentorium placement
			Meningomyelocele
Craniosynostosis	Early surgical intervention reduces or prevents serious physical, social, and neuropsychological problems	Premature fusion of cranial sutures; may be complete or partial	Misshapen skull
			May see mild hydrocephalus
	Cranial nerve dysfunction		Microcephaly
			Abnormal cephalic index
Dandy-Walker malformation	Enlarged head with bulging posterior fossa	Intracranial cystic mass (dilatation of the fourth ventricle) due to multifactorial causes, including abnormal development of the roof of the fourth ventricle, the cerebellar vermis, or genetic syndromes	Enlarged retrocerebellar cyst contiguous with fourth ventricle
	Fetal death is common		2° hydrocephalus (third and lateral ventricles)
			Elevation of tentorium and splaying of cerebellar hemispheres

Fetal cranial, spinal, and CNS abnormalities
(CONTINUED)

DISEASE PROCESS	CLINICAL, LABORATORY, AND RELATED FINDINGS	ETIOLOGY	ULTRASOUND FINDINGS
Encephalocele	↑ AFP ↑ ACE Associated with hindbrain malformations; may form part of Meckel's syndrome	Symmetric: bony defect in cranial vault (usually midline occipital) Asymmetric: amniotic band Transient pleural effusion may originate from fetal infection or brief fetal cardiac failure	Associated with ventriculomegaly and polyhydramnios Meninges with or without brain tissue bulge out of spinal defect; cystic or complex appearance; usually occurs in occiput region Fetal hydrops (peritoneal accumulation of fluid)
Holoprosencephaly		Cerebral malformations resulting from incomplete division of forebrain into two cerebral hemispheres	Intracranial midline cystic mass Absence of falx and corpus callosum

DISEASE PROCESS	CLINICAL, LABORATORY, AND RELATED FINDINGS	ETIOLOGY	ULTRASOUND FINDINGS
		Occurs sporadically or as chromosomal abnormality such as trisomy 13	Fused thalami differentiates condition from hydranencephaly, subarachnoid cyst, or posterior fossa cyst
ALOBAR	Most severe form		Fetal head enlarged
	Facial and maxillary clefts are generally present		Minimal amount of cerebral tissue visualized peripherally on floor of anterior cranial fossa
	Infants rarely survive first year of life		Hypotelorism
	Infants occasionally have cyclops		
SEMILOBAR	Less severe form		Characterized by a single large, central ventricle
	Infants have cleft palate and lip		More cerebral tissue present
			Occipital lobe tissue may be present

DISEASE PROCESS	CLINICAL, LABORATORY, AND RELATED FINDINGS	ETIOLOGY	ULTRASOUND FINDINGS
Fetal cranial, spinal, and CNS abnormalities, *Holoprosencephaly (CONTINUED)*			
LOBAR	Mildest form		Fetal head not enlarged
	Usually no facial abnormalities		Slightly dilated lateral ventricles
	Mental retardation		Absence of cavum septi pellucidi
			Associated with:
			• Absent or hypoplastic cerebellar vermis
			• Agenesis of corpus callosum
Hydranencephaly	Cerebrum entirely replaced by fluid (CSF)	Multiple causes described:	Large fluid-filled fetal cranium
			Absence of cerebral mantle

DISEASE PROCESS	CLINICAL, LABORATORY, AND RELATED FINDINGS	ETIOLOGY	ULTRASOUND FINDINGS
	Poor prognosis	• Occlusion of internal carotid arteries, causing necrosis of developing cerebral hemispheres	Brain stem, basal ganglia, and thalami visualized
	Most die within first year	• Infection	Falx usually intact
		• Syndromic	
		Skull and meninges normal	
		Cerebellum and midbrain intact	
Hydrocephalus	Occurs 0.5–3.0 times per 1000 live births with varying degrees of neurologic impairment	A progressive ↑ in volume of ventricles 2° to a relative obstruction of CSF under pressure; may be partial or complete obstruction	Ventriculomegaly, as evidenced by atria measuring >10 mm
	↑ head size with continuing ↑ in circumference	Secondary to:	Depending on etiology, can be unilateral or bilateral
	Increased intracranial pressure	▶	Choroid plexus, thickness appears relatively decreased as ventriculomegaly increases
	▶		▶

DISEASE PROCESS	CLINICAL, LABORATORY, AND RELATED FINDINGS	ETIOLOGY	ULTRASOUND FINDINGS
Fetal cranial, spinal, and CNS abnormalities, *Hydrocephalus* *(CONTINUED)*	Postbirth: Headache Vomiting Variable reduction in the level of consciousness	• Aqueductal stenosis • Hemorrhage • Infection • Intracranial mass In association with other anomalies: • Dandy-Walker malformation • Arnold-Chiari malformation • Arachnoid cysts • AV malformation • Encephalocele • Overproduction of CSF from choroid plexus papilloma	Posterior horn increases first; anterior horn increases last >70% have associated anomalies of CNS, renal, and cardiac origin Stable and V-P shunted cerebrovascular flow patterns have ↓ resistance
Kleeblattschädel *(cloverleaf skull)*	Uniformly lethal Infants have associated congenital abnormalities (e.g., skeletal dysplasia)	Craniosynostosis of only coronal and lambdoidal sutures	Delayed growth of BPD early in pregnancy Cloverleaf-shaped head May see hydrocephalus

DISEASE PROCESS	CLINICAL, LABORATORY, AND RELATED FINDINGS	ETIOLOGY	ULTRASOUND FINDINGS
			Partial falx may be identified
Meckel Gruber syndrome	Lethal	Autosomal recessive without carrier expression; karyotype is normal	Encephalocele
	Infant may have:		Polydactyly
	• Enlarged abdomen		Bilateral renal cystic dysplasia
	• Polydactyly	Recurrence risk for each subsequent pregnancy is 25%	Two components must be present to make diagnosis
	• Ambiguous genitalia		
	• Microencephaly		Oligohydramnios
	• Occipital encephalocele		Ventriculomegaly
	• Cleft lip, palate		Microcephaly
	Occurs equally in males and females		
Microcephaly	Mental restriction	Rubella infection	
	Small brain in a small skull	Cytomegalovirus infection	
	Must be certain of dates to diagnose	Toxoplasmosis infection	
		▶	

OBSTETRICS-GYNECOLOGY

DISEASE PROCESS	CLINICAL, LABORATORY, AND RELATED FINDINGS	ETIOLOGY	ULTRASOUND FINDINGS
Fetal cranial, spinal, and CNS abnormalities, *(CONTINUED)* *Microcephaly*		Severe irradiation	Demonstrates impairment of head growth BPD and HC by ≥3 standard deviations below normal AC and femur length
		Chronic maternal mercury poisoning	Serial examinations necessary
		Maternal alcoholism	
		Autosomal recessive condition	
Spinal dysraphism	Neural tube defect	Failure of neural fold fusion	Polyhydramnios
		Multifactorial	Associated with rentriculomegaly
		May be spontaneous, or may be due to genetic (associated with trisomy 18) or environmental factors such as insufficient folic acid	

DISEASE PROCESS	CLINICAL, LABORATORY, AND RELATED FINDINGS	ETIOLOGY	ULTRASOUND FINDINGS
MENINGOCELE/ MYELOMENINGOCELE	↑ MSAFP ↑ amniotic fluid ↑ AFP ↑ ACE	Results in spina bifida with herniation of meninges and/or neural tissue through bony defect	Widening of posterior ossification centers Complex, primarily cystic mass protruding from defect site; lack of normal skin covering
SPINA BIFIDA	Associated with meningocele, myelomeningocele May have ↑ AFP, (+) and acetylcholinesterase if defect is open	Spinal dysraphism due to abnormal or incomplete fusion of neural arches Lesion may be opened or closed	Coronal, sagittal, and transverse views of spine demonstrate splaying of lateral ossification centers; posterior elements may be deviated Skin may or may not appear intact at location of defect
Teratoma	↑ AFP ▶		Fetal head enlargement ▶

OBSTETRICS-GYNECOLOGY

DISEASE PROCESS	CLINICAL, LABORATORY, AND RELATED FINDINGS	ETIOLOGY	ULTRASOUND FINDINGS
Fetal cranial, spinal, and CNS abnormalities, *Teratoma (CONTINUED)*	Has potential to become malignant, especially if solid, but usually is histologically benign Prognosis dependent on size of lesion and amount of brain destruction	Congenital tumor involving a combination of germ layers in totally unorganized pattern	Midline lesion mass can appear predominantly cystic or solid, but most often is complex, primarily solid; may see areas of calcification May cause hydrocephalus due to mass compression Tumors range in size from small to very large
Fetal kidney abnormalities			
Agenesis, bilateral renal	Occurs in 1–4 infants per 10,000 births	Failure of ureteric bud to develop off mesonephric duct	Bilateral absence of kidneys Oligohydramnios Pulmonary hypoplasia

DISEASE PROCESS	CLINICAL, LABORATORY, AND RELATED FINDINGS	ETIOLOGY	ULTRASOUND FINDINGS
	Associated with facial deformities, hypertelorism, low-set ears, parrot beak nose, limb abnormalities		Absence of fetal bladder
Hydronephrosis	Most common fetal anomaly	Physiologic when <10 mm in AP diameter	Patient may have oligohydramnios (if bilateral) or normal fluid (if unilateral)
	Possible dysplasia and reduced future renal function dependent on degree of obstruction and time of onset	Ureteropelvic junction (most common for unilateral)	Anechoic renal sinus splayed, depending on degree of pelvic dilatation
		Posterior urethral valves (bilateral)	▶
		Urethral stenosis (bilateral)	
		Outlet obstruction (bilateral)	
		Ectopic ureterocele (usually unilateral)	

OBSTETRICS-GYNECOLOGY

DISEASE PROCESS	CLINICAL, LABORATORY, AND RELATED FINDINGS	ETIOLOGY	ULTRASOUND FINDINGS
Fetal kidney abnormalities, *Hydronephrosis* *(CONTINUED)*			May see bilateral dilatation of ureters if associated with urethral stenosis, posterior urethral valves, or outlet obstruction
			May see unilateral ureteral dilatation if associated with ectopic ureterocele
Hypoplastic kidney	Associated with other fetal anomalies	Failure of kidneys to develop to normal size	Unilateral or (less commonly) bilateral
			Small kidney; may be difficult to find
			Patient may have oligohydramnios (if bilateral)
			Contralateral kidney may be hypertrophied (if unilateral)

DISEASE PROCESS	CLINICAL, LABORATORY, AND RELATED FINDINGS	ETIOLOGY	ULTRASOUND FINDINGS
Infantile polycystic kidney disease	Associated with liver fibrosis, or with impaired or absent renal function	Autosomal recessive polycystic kidney disease	Oligohydramnios
			"Cysts" not seen
	Associated with Meckel's syndrome, cleft palate, microcephaly, and ambiguous genitalia	Cystic dilatation of the collecting tubules	Bilateral, enlarged, hyperechoic kidneys due to interfaces of the many microscopic cysts
Mesoblastic nephroma	No specific findings	Rare congenital kidney tumor	Solid, coarse, echogenic focal mass
	Better prognosis than classical Wilms' tumor		May contain cystic components
Multicystic dysplastic kidney	May be associated with ureteral atresia	Dysplastic condition resulting from pelvoinfundibular atresia with associated proximal ureteral atresia occurring at 8–10 weeks of embryonal stage	Usually unilateral (80%); may be bilateral (lethal)
		▶	Contralateral kidney is normal when unilateral
			▶

OBSTETRICS-GYNECOLOGY

DISEASE PROCESS	CLINICAL, LABORATORY, AND RELATED FINDINGS	ETIOLOGY	ULTRASOUND FINDINGS
Fetal kidney abnormalities, *Multicystic dysplastic kidney (CONTINUED)*		No familial incidence	Enlarged kidney with many well-encapsulated cysts varying in size and location within the distorted renal parenchyma
			Absence of connection between cystic components
Prune belly (Eagle-Barrett) syndrome	Hypotonic abdominal wall muscles	Associated with urethral displacement, obstruction, or malformation	Oligohydramnios
	Associated with dilatation of bladder resulting in:	Sporadic occurrence	Bilateral hydronephrosis (gross or mild)
	• Cryptorchidism in males (a massively distended bladder prevents testicular descent)		Bladder and ureter markedly dilated
	• Small thorax with flared ribs		Massive abdominal circumference with small thorax
	• Persistent urachal anomalies		
	Fetus may have imperforate anus		

DISEASE PROCESS	CLINICAL, LABORATORY, AND RELATED FINDINGS	ETIOLOGY	ULTRASOUND FINDINGS
Fetal pelvic abnormalities			
Hydrocele	Not significant if found in utero as isolated finding	Persistent processus vaginalis; fluid collects between tunica vaginalis layers	Male; clearly distinguishable as fluid surrounding testes within sac
Hydrometrocolpos	Findings disappear spontaneously after delivery	Maternal hormones cross placenta, stimulate accumulation of cervical and vaginal secretions in uterus and vagina	Usually cystic structure seen posterior to bladder due to fluid filling uterus and vagina
Ovarian cysts	More frequent in association with maternal diabetes Usually functional due to maternal secretion ▶	Rare Occur due to influence of maternal hormones	Usually simple cysts or serous cystadenoma May be septated ▶

DISEASE PROCESS	CLINICAL, LABORATORY, AND RELATED FINDINGS	ETIOLOGY	ULTRASOUND FINDINGS
Fetal pelvic abnormalities, *Ovarian cysts* *(CONTINUED)*	Regress after birth		May be hemorrhagic May be seen in abdomen outside of pelvis Sonographic differentials: • Choledochal cyst • Mesenteric cyst
Fetal skeletal abnormalities			
Achondrogenesis	Lethal No biochemical abnormalities Extreme micromelia Macrocrania Severe pulmonary hypoplasia	Autosomal recessive Severe form of chondrodystrophy, in which abnormal endochondral bone formation results in dwarfism Multiple classifications and inheritance patterns	Polyhydramnios is common Marked limb shortening (micromelia) Marked chest narrowing ↓ skeletal echogenicity Large head May see ventriculomegaly

DISEASE PROCESS	CLINICAL, LABORATORY, AND RELATED FINDINGS	ETIOLOGY	ULTRASOUND FINDINGS
Achondroplasia	Affects cartilaginous growth and epiphyses	Autosomal dominant (20%) or spontaneous mutation (80%)	
	Most common form of congenital bone disturbance present from birth	Spontaneous mutation results in anomalous cartilage growth	
HETEROZYGOUS		Both or one parent (heterozygote)	Short, bowed limbs
			Abdomen and chest moderately narrowed
			Protuberant forehead
			Increased BPD and HC
HOMOZYGOUS	Lethal condition	Both parents contribute genetically	Short, bowed limbs
	Hypoplastic lungs result in death		Thoracic narrowing
			▶

DISEASE PROCESS	CLINICAL, LABORATORY, AND RELATED FINDINGS	ETIOLOGY	ULTRASOUND FINDINGS
Fetal skeletal abnormalities, *Achondroplasia,* HOMOZYGOUS *(CONTINUED)*			Appreciable head-to-body disproportion Enlarged head
Hypophosphatasia	Defective mineralization, evidenced by low serum alkaline phosphatase	Abnormal reduction in the activity of alkaline phosphatase of body skeleton Autosomal recessive	Head: very thin appearance of skull interface due to poor mineralization; collapsed sutures are sometimes seen Ribs: thin, poorly visualized Spine: thin, poorly visualized Limbs: short, thin, ribbon-like appearance with fractures
Osteogenesis imperfecta	Affects fetus in utero; fractures occur before or during birth and infant is fragile after birth	Short limb dysplasia due to genetically based collagen disorders	All types have reduced visualization of cranium and long bones

DISEASE PROCESS	CLINICAL, LABORATORY, AND RELATED FINDINGS	ETIOLOGY	ULTRASOUND FINDINGS
	Parents usually are normal	Extreme skeletal bone demineralization	Thorax may appear somewhat collapsed
	Calvarium poorly mineralized; confirmed by radiograph		Multiple fractures may be seen late in pregnancy
TYPE I	Blue sclera	Autosomal dominant	Head is normal in size
			May see mild bowing of the limbs
TYPE II	Blue sclera	Autosomal recessive (has subclassifications)	Head: thin, often with collapsed cranium
	Lethal		Chest: fractures of the ribs
			Spine: questionable fractures
			Limbs: short, broad, angulated, with fractures; femurs tend to be broad, with marked bowing

OBSTETRICS-GYNECOLOGY

DISEASE PROCESS	CLINICAL, LABORATORY, AND RELATED FINDINGS	ETIOLOGY	ULTRASOUND FINDINGS
Fetal skeletal abnormalities, *Osteogenesis imperfecta* (*CONTINUED*)			
TYPE III	Normal sclera Height compromised	Autosomal recessive	Head: thin, but not as much as in Type II Chest: occasional rib fractures Limbs: fractures possible, broad bones, mild bowing, slightly short
TYPE IV	Normal sclera	Autosomal dominant (most mild form)	Head: normal size Chest: occasional rib fractures Limbs: bowing and occasional fractures may be seen

DISEASE PROCESS	CLINICAL, LABORATORY, AND RELATED FINDINGS	ETIOLOGY	ULTRASOUND FINDINGS
Thanatophoric dysplasia	Low L/S ratio	Chondrodystrophy	Polyhydramnios
	Lethal	Sporadic form of short-limbed dysplasia	Enlarged head appears asymmetric
		More commonly affects males	Prominent forehead (frontal bossing)
			Ventriculomegaly
			Marked thoracic narrowing
			Marked micromelia with ↑ soft tissue thickness
Trisomies			
Trisomy 13	Occurs in 1:5000 live births	Associated with advanced age, usually nondisjunction at first or second meiotic division; results in extra copy of chromosome 13	Holoprosencephaly (60–70%)
	Congenital heart disease is common; 50% die at birth		Midline facial defects
	▶		Polydactyly (50%)
			▶

DISEASE PROCESS	CLINICAL, LABORATORY, AND RELATED FINDINGS	ETIOLOGY	ULTRASOUND FINDINGS
Trisomies, *Trisomy 13* (CONTINUED)	Dysmorphic features: • Hypotelorism • Microphthalmia • Cleft lip and palate • Clenched fists • Abnormal ears • Prominent heels • Single palmar creases		Omphalocele Polycystic kidneys Heart defects (90%) Polyhydramnios, dependent on other findings
Trisomy 18	Occurs in 1:3000 live births 95% affected fetuses abort spontaneously Low birth weight Cardiac abnormalities Renal abnormalities	Associated with advanced maternal age, usually nondisjunction at first or second meiotic division; results in extra copy of chromosome 18	Polyhydramnios, dependent on other findings IUGR Clenched fist with overlapping index and fifth fingers Club feet or rocker bottom feet

DISEASE PROCESS	CLINICAL, LABORATORY, AND RELATED FINDINGS	ETIOLOGY	ULTRASOUND FINDINGS
	Dysmorphic features: • Prominent occiput • Micrognathia • Low-set, malformed ears • Clenched hands with overlapping index and fifth fingers • Rocker bottom feet • Single palmar creases		Umbilical, inguinal, or diaphragmatic hernia Cardiac defects Micrognathia
Trisomy 21	Associated with: • Abnormal triple screen • Congenital heart disease • Biliary, esophageal, duodenal atresias ▶	Trisomy 21 Overall risk is 1:660 live births Increases to 1:250 for women aged 35–39 and to 1:80 for those over 40	No specific findings are diagnostic May see: • Polyhydramnios, dependent on other findings ▶

OBSTETRICS-GYNECOLOGY

DISEASE PROCESS	CLINICAL, LABORATORY, AND RELATED FINDINGS	ETIOLOGY	ULTRASOUND FINDINGS
Trisomies, *Trisomy 21* *(CONTINUED)*	• Renal anomalies • Imperforate anus • Decreased AFP in 20% of patients under age 35 • Flat nasal profile • Joint hyperflexibility • Slanted palpebral fissures • Anomalous auricles • Pelvic dysplasia • Hypotonia • Brachycephaly		• Fetal heart abnormalities (VSD, endocardial cushion defects) • Renal pyelectasis • Duodenal atresia • Thickened nuchal fold (>6 mm) • Expected FL:actual FL <.91 • Expected HL:actual HL <.90 • Hypoplasia of middle phalanx of fifth digit • ↑ echogenic small bowel

GYNECOLOGY

Adenomyosis	Characteristically found in older, multiparous patients Hypermenorrhea	Endometrial glands and stroma found within uterus at least 2.5 mm from basalis layer of endometrium	Hypoechoic to hyperechoic local enlargement of myometrium; more typically in posterior aspect of uterus

DISEASE PROCESS	CLINICAL, LABORATORY, AND RELATED FINDINGS	ETIOLOGY	ULTRASOUND FINDINGS
	Dysmenorrhea		Irregularly shaped uterus with displacement of endometrium
	Clinically enlarged uterus		High-resistance flow; rarely will color flow demonstrate peripheral feeding arteries
	No significant lab findings		
Asherman's syndrome	May be asymptomatic	Mechanical trauma to endometrium during pregnancy, postpartum, or during abortal curettage resulting in extensive adhesions and adherence of uterine walls	Normal uterus without endometrial canal visualized
	Hypomenorrhea or amenorrhea since treatment or procedure		May see hematometra or hematosalpinx if adhesions in cervix cause stenosis of cervix
	Dysmenorrhea		Anechoic endometrial canal
	Characteristic findings on hysterosalpingogram (multiple synechiae)		
Brenner tumor	Relatively uncommon; <2% all ovarian neoplasms ▶		

OBSTETRICS-GYNECOLOGY

DISEASE PROCESS	CLINICAL, LABORATORY, AND RELATED FINDINGS	ETIOLOGY	ULTRASOUND FINDINGS
Brenner tumor *(CONTINUED)*	May have abnormal vaginal bleeding	Benign epithelial cell "nests" scattered throughout dense stroma with large, fibrotic component	Solid ovarian lesion
	Usually appears after menopause		<6 cm
	Clinically similar to fibroma		Unilateral, although 6.5% are bilateral
	May be accompanied by Meigs' syndrome		Well encapsulated
Cervical cancer	Childbearing to postmenopausal age group	Cervical epithelial neoplasia	Usually appears normal in early stages
	(+) Pap smear		Enlarged lower uterine segment with distorted echogenicity of cervix area
	First symptom is thin, watery, sometimes blood-tinged vaginal discharge		May see hematometra due to buildup of fluid as a result of stenotic cervix
	Universal symptom is intermittent, painless, abnormal intermenstrual bleeding		

DISEASE PROCESS	CLINICAL, LABORATORY, AND RELATED FINDINGS	ETIOLOGY	ULTRASOUND FINDINGS
	Stenotic cervical lesion may cause hematometra/pyometra		In later stages, may see secondary hydronephrosis due to ureteral obstruction or retroperitoneal lymphadenopathy
Cystadenoma			
Mucinous	Age group 20–50 yrs	Less active proliferation of epithelial neoplasm than serous type	Unilateral usually
	One of the most common epithelial tumors		More loculations than serous type, with thin, opaque septa
	10% malignant (usually after menopause)		Very large (15–20 cm)
	Benign cyst with sticky, gelatinous mucin contents and multilocular daughter cells		May see fluid-fluid levels or fluid-debris levels separated by septa within mass
Serous	Rapidly growing ▶		Smoothly rounded lesion ▶

OBSTETRICS-GYNECOLOGY

DISEASE PROCESS	CLINICAL, LABORATORY, AND RELATED FINDINGS	ETIOLOGY	ULTRASOUND FINDINGS
Cystadenoma, *Serous* (*CONTINUED*)	30% are frank serous cystadenocarcinomas; ↑ CA 125 in 82% with epithelial ovarian CA	Derived from epithelial cell covering the ovary; occasionally, papillary projections may proliferate	70% are unilateral
			Usually unilocular, pedunculated
	One of the most common epithelial tumors; comprises 30% of all ovarian neoplasms	Comprises 30% of all ovarian neoplasms	Thin-walled
			May contain low-level echoes due to debris or papillary projections
	Age group 20–50 yrs		May be enlarged up to 20 cm
	Representative calcium deposits found on pathology within stroma or connective tissue core or papillary processes		Doppler impedance: • Benign, usually high • Malignant, usually low
Ectopic pregnancy			
Acute	95% implant in tube		

DISEASE PROCESS	CLINICAL, LABORATORY, AND RELATED FINDINGS	ETIOLOGY	ULTRASOUND FINDINGS
	Acute, severe, unilateral LQ pain	Pregnancy implanted in location other than endometrium	Diagnosis is pathognomonic when embryonic pole with EHM++ is seen outside endo-metrial cavity and uterus is empty
	Patient usually has small amount of intermittent abnormal bleeding	Previous Hx: • PID • Previous tubal surgery • IUD • Endometriosis	More often seen but more difficult to diagnose: • Complex solid adnexal mass • Fluid in posterior cul-de-sac
	May have palpable adnexal mass	(Note: pseudogestational sac is due to decidual reaction from another pregnancy site)	• Enlarged tube • Enlarged uterus or pseudogestational sac
	Serum β-hCG ≥6500 mIU/ml transabdominally or 1800 mIU/ml endovaginally with no IUP ▶		Color Doppler displays prominent peritrophoblastic vascular signs at "adnexal mass" periphery with low impedance signal ▶
	Serial β-hCG levels rise, but not at normal rate for IUP ▶		

OBSTETRICS-GYNECOLOGY

DISEASE PROCESS	CLINICAL, LABORATORY, AND RELATED FINDINGS	ETIOLOGY	ULTRASOUND FINDINGS
Ectopic pregnancy, *Acute (CONTINUED)*	With rupture, sudden acute pain, fainting, tachycardia, pallor, and BP drop may occur		Solid extrauterine mass; mimics abscess or acute ectopic pregnancy
Chronic	Palpable pelvic mass Patient may have recurrent intermittent fever Low or absent β-hCG	Trophoblast has insufficient hormones to maintain blood supply but enough to keep trophoblast; inflammatory response occurs	May see clot formation in the cul-de-sac
Endometrial cancer	Majority of patients are postmenopausal; median age is 60	Increased number of endometrial glands replacing normal supporting stroma due to estrogenic stimulation Biopsy is the basis of a conclusive diagnosis	Uterus may be normal or may be enlarged and lobular, with change in texture Endometrial canal may be deviated Less acoustic attenuation than with leiomyoma

DISEASE PROCESS	CLINICAL, LABORATORY, AND RELATED FINDINGS	ETIOLOGY	ULTRASOUND FINDINGS
	Postmenopausal vaginal bleeding is the most common symptom; patient may have occasional spotting, which later becomes more frequent and profuse	Premenopausal conditions increasing risk are endometrial hyperplasia, dysfunctional uterine bleeding, and polycystic ovaries	25% occur in fundus
			May see hypoechoic ring around endometrial cavity in patient who is not on hormone treatment
	Pain is not a predominant feature of clinical picture		Thickness of endometrial lining (>6 mm), with heterogeneous echo pattern
Endometrioma (focal endometriosis)	Pelvic tenderness at time of menses	Walled-off implant; most common site is ovaries	Large, discrete focal mass, which appears as a thick-walled, discrete mass with irregular borders and low-level internal echoes
	Pain may be unilateral or bilateral		
	Pain may radiate to thighs		Can be cystic, complex, or solid; bilateral or unilateral

DISEASE PROCESS	CLINICAL, LABORATORY, AND RELATED FINDINGS	ETIOLOGY	ULTRASOUND FINDINGS
Endometriosis	Undesired infertility may be clinical presenting symptom

Cyclic pain (pelvic tenderness just prior to and during menses); pain not necessarily related to degree of disease but rather to location of implants; dyspareunia; dyschezia; patient in middle to late 20s; 20–30% of the population affected

No significant lab findings | Presence of endometrial tissue in abnormal locations outside uterus, either diffusely throughout pelvis and at distant sites or focally

Occurs most commonly in ovarian wall, tubes, broad ligament, posterior cul-de-sac, rectovaginal septum

Color Doppler with variable peripheral flow seen around mass; ↓ to ↑ resistance, depending on blood resorption and menstrual cycle phase. In proliferative phase, higher resistance than in secretory phase | Diffuse: may see nonspecific contour changes of pelvic structures and loss of normal tissue planes |

DISEASE PROCESS	CLINICAL, LABORATORY, AND RELATED FINDINGS	ETIOLOGY	ULTRASOUND FINDINGS
Fibroma	Palpable mass (varies in size from nodules to melon size)	Ovarian stromal origin; pure fibrous connective tissue	90% are unilateral
		Nonfunctioning	Solid mass with attenuation
	Associated with Meigs' syndrome in up to 3% of cases	Benign	Usually pedunculated
Germ cell tumors			
Cystic teratoma (dermoid)	Usually asymptomatic	Neoplasm derived from all three germ cell layers within and around ovary	Complex, moderate-sized mass usually pedunculated, with thick, irregular walls
	Occurs at any age but usually <20 yrs		May be cystic, complex, or solid
	If torsion or infarction occurs, patient presents with acute pelvic pain and N/V	Bulk of cyst is usually fatty, semi-solid sebaceous material, collection of matted hair and well-formed teeth	Generally, dense pelvic echoes produce acoustic attenuation or shadowing
	Insidious ↑ abdominal girth or adnexal fullness		▶
	▶		

DISEASE PROCESS	CLINICAL, LABORATORY, AND RELATED FINDINGS	ETIOLOGY	ULTRASOUND FINDINGS
Germ cell tumors, *Cystic teratoma (dermoid)* (*CONTINUED*)	If cyst is ruptured, patient may have peritonitis		Solid-fluid or fluid-fluid with septal pattern is most suggestive of teratoma
			75–85% are unilateral
Dysgerminoma	Occurs at all ages	Neoplasm of undifferentiated germ cells; malignant	85% are unilateral
	Peak occurrence in second or third decade of life	Ovarian counterpart of testicular seminoma	Solid mass
	Rapidly growing palpable mass	Relatively rare; <5% of ovarian malignancies	Ranges from a nodule to a mass large enough to fill the abdomen (less often malignant if <10 cm)
	75% 5-yr survival rate		
	May be benign but return as malignant		Occasionally cystic within due to necrosis
	Pure dysgerminomas do not produce hCG or AFP		
Gestational trophoblastic disease	Mean incidence 1:1000	Fertilization of ovum with no active chromosome material;	Color Doppler: uterus usually exhibits low-impedance, high diastolic flow

DISEASE PROCESS	CLINICAL, LABORATORY, AND RELATED FINDINGS	ETIOLOGY	ULTRASOUND FINDINGS
		then sperm chromosome reduplicates	
Choriocarcinoma	Discovery of metastatis (lung, vagina, cervix, vulva, liver, brain) following evacuation of mole, hysterectomy with continued uterine bleeding, or normal pregnancy

Spread to liver, lung/brain

↑↑ β-hCG | Aggressive malignant neoplasm of epithelial trophoblastic origin; spreads hematogenously

Rare

Absence of villous structures | Persistent, enlarged, bilateral theca-lutein cysts, 4–8 cm

Focal, irregular echogenic region within uterine myometrium surrounded by irregular anechoic areas (corresponding to myometrial hemorrhage)

Metastases to liver appear as echogenic foci |
| Fetus with complete mole | Uterus large for dates

FHM (+++) | Twin gestation
▶ | Normal placenta and fetus seen separate from molar tissue with characteristic molar appearance |

DISEASE PROCESS	CLINICAL, LABORATORY, AND RELATED FINDINGS	ETIOLOGY	ULTRASOUND FINDINGS
Gestational trophoblastic disease, *Fetus with complete mole (CONTINUED)*		Theoretically, one is 1st trimester embryonic demise that develops into mole	
Hydatidiform mole, complete	Vaginal bleeding	Abnormal proliferation of trophoblastic tissue	Appears as solid mass; ↑↑ echogenicity; very transonic, with multiple diffuse intraplacental anechoic lesions measuring 2–10 mm each
	Pregnancy test always positive	Mole usually has some chromosomal deviation; diagnosis based on histology	
	Pregnancy symptoms, which may include:		
	• Gravid hyperemesis	XX karyotype, majority	30–50% of cases have bilateral theca lutein cysts that can become very large (>6 cm) and septated; may persist for 2–4 mos after mole evacuation
	• Enlarged uterus	XY karyotype, rare	
	• Large for dates	20% are followed by invasive sequelae	
	• No FHT		
	• Unilateral or bilateral adnexal masses		No evidence of fetal tissue
	Markedly ↑ serum or urine hCG (up to 400,000 mIU/ml)		

DISEASE PROCESS	CLINICAL, LABORATORY, AND RELATED FINDINGS	ETIOLOGY	ULTRASOUND FINDINGS
	Preeclampsia prior to 24 wks (key finding)		May see focal areas of hypoechoic pattern due to confluent hemorrhage
	If patient tests positive, ches: x-ray rules out lung metastases		
Hydatidiform mole, partial	Mother may present with preeclampsia	Polyploidal genotype typically triploidy; fertilization of a normal haploid ovum by two normal haploid sperm; or fertilization of a normal ovum by an abnormal diploid sperm (mosaic pattern)	Vesicle filled uterus in association with some fetal structures with membrane present
	Uterine enlargement less common		May see bilaterally enlarged ovaries with many large cysts (theca-lutein cysts)
	↑↑↑ hCG	Almost always benign	
Leiomyoma (fibroid)	Most common uterine tumor	Initially, localized proliferation of smooth muscle cells and connective tissue	Intrauterine solid mass(es); usually multiple; variable in size
	Patient is usually over 30 yrs of age ▶	▶	Uterus enlarged, lobulated ▶

DISEASE PROCESS	CLINICAL, LABORATORY, AND RELATED FINDINGS	ETIOLOGY	ULTRASOUND FINDINGS
Leiomyoma (fibroid) *(CONTINUED)*	Increases in size with pregnancy and may degenerate	Eventually, degenerative central area of necrosis or hemorrhage	Solid heterogeneous echo pattern
	Develops in 20–30% of all women, more frequently in black women	Malignant potential is minimal	May attenuate sound
	Patient is usually asymptomatic but may have pain, congestive or pressure symptoms, abnormal increased bleeding; symptoms regress after menopause		Endometrial canal may be deviated or obscured by tumor(s)
			Decreased echoes within mass core due to necrosis may be seen
	No significant lab findings		Variable levels of echogenicity, ranging from hypoechoic to complex
			May be within uterine wall (intramural), subserosal, or pedunculated

DISEASE PROCESS	CLINICAL, LABORATORY, AND RELATED FINDINGS	ETIOLOGY	ULTRASOUND FINDINGS
			Cannot rule out malignant neoplastic process from ultrasound findings
			May calcify with or without acoustic shadowing
			Color usually demonstrates peripheral feeding arteries with low resistance, high diastolic flow; mean RI = 0.54
Meigs' syndrome	Ascites and pleural effusion, usually in association with palpable ovarian fibroma	Transudate of extracellular fluid and leakage through thin fibroma capsule; result of local peritoneal irritation	Four characteristics:
			• Ovarian mass (solid)
	History of nonmalignant tumor		• Ascites
	Chest x-ray demonstrates pleural effusion	Pleural effusion from excessive abdominal fluid passing through lymphatics of the diaphragm	• Pleural effusion
	▶		• Resolves following surgery

OBSTETRICS-GYNECOLOGY

DISEASE PROCESS	CLINICAL, LABORATORY, AND RELATED FINDINGS	ETIOLOGY	ULTRASOUND FINDINGS
Meigs' syndrome (CONTINUED)	KUB demonstrates abdominal mass with accompanying ascites		
	Disappears completely and permanently following removal of tumor		
Ovarian cysts			
Corpus luteum cyst	Usually asymptomatic	Corpus luteum of menstruation arises as a result of hemorrhage within a persistent, mature corpus luteum	Anechoic single cyst, usually about 2 cm; can grow to >5 cm
	Produces menstrual irregularities if persistent		Smooth-walled with posterior acoustic enhancement
	Pelvic and lower abdominal pain (usually unilateral)	Corpus luteum of pregnancy is associated with maintenance of first 10 wks of pregnancy	May see free-fluid in cul-de-sac if rupture occurs
	May rupture, producing acute surgical emergency		May appear as a complex adnexal mass, depending on state of hemorrhage
	Can be associated with early IUP and ↑ β-hCG values		

DISEASE PROCESS	CLINICAL, LABORATORY, AND RELATED FINDINGS	ETIOLOGY	ULTRASOUND FINDINGS
			Corpus luteum of pregnancy measures up to 5 cm
			Color Doppler exhibits low resistance, high diastolic flow
Follicular cyst	May be associated with menstrual irregularity if persistent	Unruptured dominant follicle fails to ovulate and remains active but immature; alternatively, less-stimulated follicles fail to undergo normal regression	Cysts usually remain small (1–1.5 cm) but can grow to 5 cm
	May result in increased estrogen production if persistent		Usually multiple
	Usually disappears spontaneously, either by slow resorption of fluid or by sudden rupture (which may produce transient acute or chronic intermittent lower abdominal pain)		Ovary remains within normal size limits and is otherwise homogeneous in echogenicity
			Cysts are thin-walled, unilocular

OBSTETRICS-GYNECOLOGY

DISEASE PROCESS	CLINICAL, LABORATORY, AND RELATED FINDINGS	ETIOLOGY	ULTRASOUND FINDINGS
Ovarian cysts *(CONTINUED)*			
Polycystic ovaries	Appears after menarche	Noncongenital anomaly related to self-perpetuating cycle of irregularities in LH, FSH, and estrogen secretion (as described)	25% of patients have normal-sized ovaries, in which peripheral follicles are visualized on serial exams and will persist
	No ovulation due to ↓ FSH		
	Patient is infertile		70% of patients have bilateral enlarged ovaries (up to 3× normal size)
	Hirsutism (seen in 50–60% of patients with polycystic ovary disease)	Rarely, involves pituitary dysfunction	
	Obesity		Three categories of findings:
	Menstrual irregularities (oligomenorrhea)		• Bilateral discrete ovarian cysts found peripherally; 2–6 mm
	Decreased FSH, steady LH stimulate excess ovarian androgen production (serum testosterone and DHEAS)		• Ovaries hypoechoic to uterus • Ovaries isoechoic to uterus

DISEASE PROCESS	CLINICAL, LABORATORY, AND RELATED FINDINGS	ETIOLOGY	ULTRASOUND FINDINGS
	No fluctuation in estrogen levels		
Theca-lutein cyst	Increased serum β-hCG	Rarely arises independently; vast majority occur in association with ↑ levels of hCG	Bilateral thin-walled cystic masses
	Usually associated with hydatidiform mole and choriocarcinoma		May attain sizes ranging from 2.5–3.0 cm to 20.0 cm
	Regression with removal of mole or trophoblastic lesion occurs within 2–4 mos	May be associated with infertility drug hyperstimulation	Multiple septa
Ovarian carcinoma	Mean age 52 yrs	Most common lethal gynecologic malignancy	Complex, primarily solid adnexal mass; ascites common
	Vague symptoms	Epithelial origin; undifferentiated cells	Low impedance flow carries ↑ concerns for malignancy when RI < 0.40
	Pelvic pressure, pain		
	GI symptoms		

DISEASE PROCESS	CLINICAL, LABORATORY, AND RELATED FINDINGS	ETIOLOGY	ULTRASOUND FINDINGS
Pelvic inflammatory disease (PID)	Gonococcus resides in tubes; chlamydia resides in endocervix and produces increasing amounts of pyometra	Variable, usually multifactorial: • Chlamydia • Gonorrhea (65–75% of cases with bacterial etiology) • Endogenous anaerobic bacteria (e.g., *Bacteroides*) • Aerobic bacteria (e.g., *Streptococcus, E. coli*) • Nonbacterial (IUD, septic abortion, etc.)	Color Doppler in PID: • Increased vascularization • Waveform patterns variable; generally low resistance to blood flow
Chronic pelvic inflammatory disease	Intractable pelvic pain May lead to infertility or ectopic pregnancy No significant lab findings	Long-standing residue of acute infection with subacute recurrence of previous PID, with subsequent adhesion of pelvic structures to each other Chronic disease may be immunologically mediated	Obliteration of the margins between the uterus and adnexa May appear as ill-defined adnexal mass with complex echogenic pattern May see peritoneal fluid

DISEASE PROCESS	CLINICAL, LABORATORY, AND RELATED FINDINGS	ETIOLOGY	ULTRASOUND FINDINGS
Endometritis	50–80% of patients are asymptomatic	Inflammation of endometrium following:	May be normal ultrasound (75%)
		• Recent C-section	Uterus enlarged (swollen)
	Patient may have:	• Abortion	May see cul-de-sac fluid
	• Vaginal discharge	• IUD perforation	Endometrium widened and
	• Urethral burning	• Retention of products of	generally inhomogeneous or
	• ↑ WBC	conception	may be very echogenic
	• ↑ Sedimentation rate	• Contamination of uterine cavity	
		by m croorganisms of vagina	May see air in endometrial
	Patient may have:	Not necessarily related to PID	cavity (due to gas-producing
	• (+) Culture for chlamydia,		infection)
	gonococcus, etc.		
	• Recent complicated abortion		May see fluid within endometrial
	• History of exposure to		cavity or may see hypoechoic
	venereal disease		halo around endometrium
	▶		(Note: should see no air 48 hrs
			after surgery)

OBSTETRICS-GYNECOLOGY

DISEASE PROCESS	CLINICAL, LABORATORY, AND RELATED FINDINGS	ETIOLOGY	ULTRASOUND FINDINGS
Pelvic inflammatory disease (PID), *Endometritis* (CONTINUED)	• Recent C-section or postpartum patient; usually spikes fever within 24 hrs after delivery (yellowish-green to black discharge is found in the lochia) Can progress to myometritis, parametritis, pelvic abscess, or peritonitis		
Pelvic abscess with peritonitis	Fitz-Hugh–Curtis syndrome (acute RUQ pain) (10%) High fever Significantly ↑ WBC (>20,000 with left shift)	Diffuse spread of purulent fluid to surrounding peritoneal cavity	Free fluid in hepatorenal space and in cul-de-sac Pelvic tissue edema and gas-forming abscesses result in loss of normal sonographic tissue planes

DISEASE PROCESS	CLINICAL, LABORATORY, AND RELATED FINDINGS	ETIOLOGY	ULTRASOUND FINDINGS
Salpingitis	Cervical tenderness	Tubes become edematous with progressive disease	Swollen tubes appear more echogenic with pyosalpinx; characteristic serpiginous shape due to edema; proximal tube tapered; sequela is anechoic as pus resorbs
	Adnexal tenderness	Purulent exudate further distends tubes(s)	
	Acute or constant dull abdominal complaint	With resolution, hydrosalpinx remains	
	May lead to abscess		
Tubo-ovarian abscess (TOA)	Febrile shaking chills (>38.3°C)	Abscess involving both tube and ovaries	Thick-walled, complex mass
	Symptoms of acute abdominal pain		Fluid in adnexa/cul-de-sac
	Leukocytosis (50%)		Debris of pyosalpinx combined with adnexal fluid makes ultrasound less specific
	↑ erythrocyte sed rate		Unilateral or bilateral
	↑ PMNs		

PROSTATE

Size variable according to life stage
- normal: 3 cm long
  2 cm AP diameter
  4 cm transverse width
- age 20–40 years: gland enlarges
- age 40–50 years: gland becomes largest

PROSTATE

212

DISEASE PROCESS	CLINICAL, LABORATORY, AND RELATED FINDINGS	ETIOLOGY	ULTRASOUND FINDINGS*
Normal		Develops from epithelial evaginations that initially appear along the pelvic-urethra during the tenth week of gestation	Appears as a homogeneous, symmetrical, medium-level structure posterior to the urinary bladder and caudal to the less echogenic seminal vesicles seen posterior, superior, and lateral to gland
			Zones surrounding ejaculatory ducts, prostatic urethra and verumontanum can be distinguished
Benign prostatic hypertrophy	May be asymptomatic Very common in men (>50%) over 50 yrs of age	Hypertrophy of the periurethral glands and distention of the acini of the glands; limited to central zone	Shape extremely variable (depending on degree of severity)

*Ultrasound findings for the prostate are by transrectal transducer cross sections.

DISEASE PROCESS	CLINICAL, LABORATORY, AND RELATED FINDINGS	ETIOLOGY	ULTRASOUND FINDINGS
	First symptom is usually dysuria in association with urinary frequency		Well-defined, smooth margins of prostate
	Eventually, complete urinary retention occurs, causing severe suprapubic pain		Prostate appears symmetric; divided into central zone and peripheral external zone
	Increase in level of PSA is variable		As hyperplasia develops, the central zone occupies more of the prostate capsule
			Echo pattern may appear heterogeneous due to: • Formation of nodules • Stones, which may or may not shadow • Areas of infarction • Ductal dilatation

BENIGN PROSTATIC HYPERTROPHY

PROSTATE

DISEASE PROCESS	CLINICAL, LABORATORY, AND RELATED FINDINGS	ETIOLOGY	ULTRASOUND FINDINGS
Carcinoma	Most common male cancer in the U.S.	Adenocarcinoma of the prostate	Prostate may appear asymmetrically enlarged
	Occurs in 12–45% of men over 50 years of age	Source occurs most often in peripheral zone	Tumor shape variable; variable echo pattern; may be hyperechoic, hypoechoic, or isoechoic to normal prostate parenchyma
	Clinical symptoms usually occur after cancer has already infiltrated locally or metastasis has begun; alternatively, found incidentally when specimens are removed for hyperplasia		May see calcifications with irregular distribution in prostate, often accompanied by diffuse, increased echoes around them due to inflammation
	Degree of ↑ PSA is variable		Color Doppler imaging may identify area of hypervascularity
			Check for gland symmetry
			Check for capsule irregularity

DISEASE PROCESS	CLINICAL, LABORATORY, AND RELATED FINDINGS	ETIOLOGY	ULTRASOUND FINDINGS
Prostatitis			
Acute	Occurs more frequently in men 20–50 yrs of age	Usually 2° to acute posterior urethritis	Prostate is enlarged and has a normal to deformed contour
	Frequency		Variable echo pattern, ranging from hypoechoic to hyperechoic
	Urgency		
	Painful urination		Size and shape return to normal following treatment, but abnormal echo pattern may remain
	Perineal and rectal pain		
	Urinary retention		
	Fever		Color Doppler indicates areas of hypervascularity
	Patient may have hematuria		
	▶		
Chronic	Occurs more frequently in older age groups	May be 2° to acute or subacute urethritis or acute prostatitis as a result of nonspecific bacteria	

PROSTATE

DISEASE PROCESS	CLINICAL, LABORATORY, AND RELATED FINDINGS	ETIOLOGY	ULTRASOUND FINDINGS
Prostatitis, *Chronic* (*CONTINUED*)	Frequency		Well-defined, normal-sized prostate or may see capsular thickening and irregularity
	Urgency		
	Painful urination		Abnormal patterns of focal masses or diffuse, heterogeneous echo pattern
	Perineal and rectal aching		
	Low back pain		May see punctate calcifications within gland (e.g., ejaculatory duct calcifications)
	Patient may have purulent discharge		

RETROPERITONEUM

RETROPERITONEUM

DISEASE PROCESS	CLINICAL, LABORATORY, AND RELATED FINDINGS	ETIOLOGY	ULTRASOUND FINDINGS
Lymphadenopathy	Degree of swelling or pain related to primary disease	Lymphoma Metastatic tumors (testicle, renal cell, uterus, cervix, etc.) Infection AIDS and AIDS-related diseases	Nodes >1 cm can be seen with high-resolution equipment; visualized in para-aortic, mesenteric, and celiac nodes Nodes appear homogeneous, hypoechoic, or anechoic, with low-level echogenicity and smooth borders (but less so than aortic aneurysm); no posterior acoustic enhancement As nodes enlarge, they may become irregular in appearance and may displace surrounding anatomy

DISEASE PROCESS	CLINICAL, LABORATORY, AND RELATED FINDINGS	ETIOLOGY	ULTRASOUND FINDINGS
			As nodes diffusely enlarge, they will create a mantle appearance over and around prevertebral vessels and may have a lobular, smooth, or scalloped appearance; if mesenteric adenopathy is also seen, the "sandwich sign" will appear
			With full bladder, may identify nodes anterior and medial to iliac vessel margins
			Retroperitoneal tumor plus ascites usually indicates seeding or invasion of peritoneal surface
			May see liver metastases

LYMPHADENOPATHY

RETROPERITONEUM

DISEASE PROCESS	CLINICAL, LABORATORY, AND RELATED FINDINGS	ETIOLOGY	ULTRASOUND FINDINGS
Masses	May see fine calcifications on x-ray	Primary tumors: • Leiomyosarcoma • Liposarcoma • Fibrosarcoma • Neuroblastoma • Rhabdomyosarcoma • Teratoma	Ill-defined, heterogeneous mass Dramatic distortion of organ anatomy, displacement or indentation of great vessel; will not be distorted when pressure is applied by the transducer May be highly echogenic May appear complex, with hypoechoic or cystic areas (due to necrosis or hemorrhage)
Retroperitoneal fibrosis	May occur in association with aortic aneurysm Patient may have hydronephrosis due to encasement of ureter	Unknown May be idiopathic, related to infiltrating neoplasm, or acute immune disease	Discrete, hypoechoic mass of smooth-contoured tissue lying anterior and lateral to great vessels

DISEASE PROCESS	CLINICAL, LABORATORY, AND RELATED FINDINGS	ETIOLOGY	ULTRASOUND FINDINGS
	Leukocytosis		Difficult to differentiate from lymphoma
	Anemia		May displace or encase great vessels, causing indentation of lumen
	Fever		

RETROPERITONEAL FIBROSIS

TESTES AND SCROTUM

Normal testis size

- 4–5 cm long
- 3 cm AP diameter
- 3 cm transverse width

Goals of ultrasound exam

- Check for size, shape, symmetry, and echo pattern of testes within scrotal sac
- Determine configuration of any abnormality
- Determine if abnormalities are intra- or extratesticular

TESTES AND SCROTUM

DISEASE PROCESS	CLINICAL, LABORATORY, AND RELATED FINDINGS	ETIOLOGY	ULTRASOUND FINDINGS
Normal		Originating from medial side of mesonephros, the male gonad is surrounded by the tunica albuginea (directly enveloping the testes) and the two layers of the tunica vaginalis (enveloping the testicular organ); these layers create the space for potential fluid accumulation	Ovoid structure beneath scrotal wall
			4.0–5.0 cm sagittal, 2.5–3.0 cm transverse width, and 3.0 cm anterior posterior diameter
			Smooth, homogeneous echo pattern; may see linear echogenicities at mediastinum
			Epididymis lies along the posterolateral wall and enlarges at the superiorly located head of the epididymis; echogenic pattern is similar to that of the testes, although the texture is more coarse; the Doppler waveform shows low impedance

DISEASE PROCESS	CLINICAL, LABORATORY, AND RELATED FINDINGS	ETIOLOGY	ULTRASOUND FINDINGS
Carcinoma			
Choriocarcinoma	Most malignant testicular tumor; least common	Nonseminomatous, usually mixed germ cell tumor	Irregular tumor; appears complex, with cystic and calcific regions (due to hemorrhage and necrosis)
	Occurs in second and third decades of life and in 1–3%	Rare	Widespread metastasis may be seen
	Fatal prognosis (100%); usually death occurs within 6 mos		
	Widespread metastases		
	Insidious onset, with painless enlargement of the testicle		
	Small, nodular, hard mass with abundant hemorrhage		
	↑ hCG (100%); commonly results in gynecomastia		

CARCINOMA

TESTES AND SCROTUM

DISEASE PROCESS	CLINICAL, LABORATORY, AND RELATED FINDINGS	ETIOLOGY	ULTRASOUND FINDINGS
Carcinoma *(CONTINUED)*			
Embryonal cell	Second most frequent type of testicular germ cell tumor	Germ cell tumor of varied histologic makeup, poorly differentiated	Usually small, hypoechoic mass compared to surrounding testicle, with areas of increased echogenicity due to calcification
	Occurs in 20–25% of cases		
	Occurs most frequently in third decade of life		Mass may invade epididymis
	Patient presents with testicular swelling and pain		Irregular borders
	May have ↑ AFP, hCG, or both		
	Variably extensive hemorrhage and necrosis		
Mixed germ cell	Occurs in second and third decades of life	Various combinations of neoplastic germ cell elements	Appears complex, with mixed solid and cystic components

DISEASE PROCESS	CLINICAL, LABORATORY, AND RELATED FINDINGS	ETIOLOGY	ULTRASOUND FINDINGS
	90% have ↑ AFP and hCG	Most frequent combination is teratoma and embryonal cell	Differentials for above lesions based on ultrasound appearance alone • Epididymitis • Spermatocele • Benign stromal tumor • Orchitis • Infarction
Seminoma	Most common primary neoplasm (30–50% of neoplasms) Usually occurs in the third to fifth decade of life Patient presents with firm, painless testicular swelling ▶	Undifferentiated germ cell tumor, including: • Typical (90% of cases) • Anaplastic • Spermatocytic • Synchiotrophoblastic giant cell	Hypoechoic lesion within surrounding testis Well demarcated, with smooth, clearly defined borders appearing round or oval May see retroperitoneal lymphadenopathy

CARCINOMA

TESTES AND SCROTUM

DISEASE PROCESS	CLINICAL, LABORATORY, AND RELATED FINDINGS	ETIOLOGY	ULTRASOUND FINDINGS
Carcinoma, *Seminoma* *(CONTINUED)*	Metastasis uncommon Good prognosis with radiation treatment ↑ hCG (10%)		
Teratoma	Accounts for <10% of primary neoplasms Occurs within the first three decades of life Hemorrhage and necrosis are not typical ↑ AFP (50%) if malignant ↑ hCG (50%)	Germ cell tumor characterized by tissue from all three germ layers Usually benign, but when occurring in adults are considered malignant; one-third metastasize, usually via lymphatic route	Complex, primarily cystic or solid, appearing within the enlarged testicle May have echogenic areas with acoustic shadow due to cartilaginous foci or bone formation

DISEASE PROCESS	CLINICAL, LABORATORY, AND RELATED FINDINGS	ETIOLOGY	ULTRASOUND FINDINGS
Epididymitis			
Acute	Acute onset of unilateral painful swelling of scrotum	Inflammation and thickening of the epididymis due to:	Enlarged epididymis, appears heterogeneous
	Malaise	• Trauma	Hypoechoic to anechoic echogenicity compared to normal
	Dysuria	• Lower urinary tract infections	
	Fever	• Gonococcus	Usually testicle appears normal, but may have focal hypoechoic areas due to focal orchitis
	↑WBC	• Chlamydia	
		• Neoplasm	
		• TB	May see associated hydrocele
		• Prostatitis	Color Doppler usually shows ↑ blood flow in epididymis and/or testis compared to other side, depending on degree of inflammation

EPIDIDYMITIS

DISEASE PROCESS	CLINICAL, LABORATORY, AND RELATED FINDINGS	ETIOLOGY	ULTRASOUND FINDINGS
Epididymitis *(CONTINUED)*			
Chronic	Slow enlargement of the scrotum occurs	*See* Epididymitis, acute, p. 229	Epididymis may appear enlarged, with diffusely inhomogeneous echogenicity and increased color flow, depending on degree of inflammation
	Patient may have hard, palpable scrotal mass with dull, aching pain		Focal or generalized thickening of epididymis is a common finding
			May see calcifications
			May see associated hydrocele
			If testes are involved, may appear inhomogeneous and irregular

DISEASE PROCESS	CLINICAL, LABORATORY, AND RELATED FINDINGS	ETIOLOGY	ULTRASOUND FINDINGS
Hernia	Most common cause of inguinal swelling	Herniation of bowel and/or omentum into the scrotal sac	Normal testicles separate from scrotal "mass" with peristalsis, which is contiguous with the inguinal canal
	Seldom associated with pain or tenderness		May be found in association with hydrocele
Hydrocele	Most common reason for painless scrotal swelling	Abnormal accumulation of serous fluid, blood, pus, or urine (usually 50–100 ml) between the parietal and visceral layers of the tunica vaginalis due to:	Anechoic collection of >2 mm of fluid surrounding the testis within the layers of the tunica vaginalis
	May be associated with pain	• Infection within the testis or epididymis	
	Patient may have history of trauma or infection	• Lymphogenous spread of disease	Because of posterior acoustic enhancement through fluid surrounding testicle, testis may seem relatively hyperechoic
		▶	▶

HYDROCELE

231

TESTES AND SCROTUM

DISEASE PROCESS	CLINICAL, LABORATORY, AND RELATED FINDINGS	ETIOLOGY	ULTRASOUND FINDINGS
Hydrocele *(CONTINUED)*		• Trauma • Neoplasm • Torsion May be idiopathic	May see debris or septa in fluid if chronic or hemorrhagic
Spermatocele	Asymptomatic Common in children Cysts contain a milky fluid when aspirated; contains nonviable sperm (if past puberty), fat, lymphocytes, and cellular debris May create "heavy" sensation in scrotum and groin May result in infertility	Retention cyst of the epididymis thought to arise from segmental obstruction in rete testes Can occur with: • Trauma • Chronic epididymitis	Typically arises near head of epididymis Usually solitary, 2- to 3-mm lesion Appears as anechoic, loculated lesion indistinguishable from hydrocele on ultrasound Color flow will detect no flow pattern

232

DISEASE PROCESS	CLINICAL, LABORATORY, AND RELATED FINDINGS	ETIOLOGY	ULTRASOUND FINDINGS
			Color Doppler will demonstrate venous flow pattern; varicocele follows course of spermatic cord into inguinal canal
Torsion	Scrotal swelling Pain	Impedance of testicular arterial supply; results in ischemia and testicular infarction	*Early:* Normal testis with detectable color flow, although may be reduced compared to other testis *Late:* Inhomogeneous testis with no detectable color flow; may have ↑ flow in twisted spermatic cord

TORSION

233

TESTES AND SCROTUM

DISEASE PROCESS	CLINICAL, LABORATORY, AND RELATED FINDINGS	ETIOLOGY	ULTRASOUND FINDINGS
Varicocele	Occurs more commonly on left side due to angle of left spermatic vein emptying into left renal vein May be asymptomatic (small varicocele)	Collection of dilated (varicose) veins of the pampiniform plexus Dilated veins may be sclerotic or thrombotic	Tortuous, ectatic veins appear as tubular, fluid-filled structures superior and sometimes posterior to the testicle

THYROID - PARATHYROID

THYROID-PARATHYROID

DISEASE PROCESS	CLINICAL, LABORATORY, AND RELATED FINDINGS	ETIOLOGY	ULTRASOUND FINDINGS
Normal	In most cases, upper margin of isthmus lies just inferior to cricoid cartilage	Originates as epithelial thickening on the pharyngeal floor	Each lobe measures: • 4–6 cm longitudinally • 1–2 cm anteroposteriorly • 2–3 cm transversely
	Lateral to glands are carotid arteries, jugular veins, and sternocleidomastoid muscles	Normally composed of tiny follicles within gland	Granular, homogeneous, medium-level echo pattern throughout bilateral lobes
			Fibrous capsule is smooth-bordered and not imaged unless thickened
			Trachea appears medially as bright reflector with acoustic reverberation artifacts

DISEASE PROCESS	CLINICAL, LABORATORY, AND RELATED FINDINGS	ETIOLOGY	ULTRASOUND FINDINGS
			Adjacent longus colli posterior, sternocleidomastoid, and strap muscles anterior and lateral to thyroid appear hypoechoic compared to the thyroid lobes
			Vascularity:
			• Carotid is medial to jugular
			• Appears anechoic
			• Appears round, with pulsations on transverse cuts
			• Appears tubular with pulsations on sagittal cuts
			• Jugular will enlarge with Valsalva maneuver
			▶

NORMAL

THYROID-PARATHYROID

DISEASE PROCESS	CLINICAL, LABORATORY, AND RELATED FINDINGS	ETIOLOGY	ULTRASOUND FINDINGS
Normal *(CONTINUED)*			With color Doppler, both the inferior and superior thyroid artery branches are seen; otherwise, glandular vascularity is minimal
			Esophagus, anteriorlateral and to left of trachea, appears as hypoechoic structure with a central echogenic center; elevates when swallowing
Adenoma			
Parathyroid	Responsible for 80% of hyperparathyroid pathologies	Benign tumor of parathyroid gland	Oval discrete lesion >5 mm; located posterior to the thyroid gland and anterior to the longus colli muscle, medial to the location of the neurovascular muscle
	Occurs slilighty more often in males than in females	May be primary (resulting from hyperfunctioning of all glands)	
	Usually affects one gland		

DISEASE PROCESS	CLINICAL, LABORATORY, AND RELATED FINDINGS	ETIOLOGY	ULTRASOUND FINDINGS
	↑ serum calcium ↓ serum phosphate	May be secondary (resulting from poor renal function or rickets)	Appears anechoic to hypoechoic compared to thyroid tissue Usually solitary Sonographic differentials: • Hyperplasia • Carcinoma
Thyroid	Most common solid nodule Can undergo cystic degeneration Rarely extends beyond the thyroid capsule	Benign solid tumors of the thyroid resulting from production of glandular acini within thyroid stroma	A broad spectrum of appearances, ranging from predominantly anechoic to complex to completely hyperechoic (depending on whether degeneration has occurred) Most are well circumscribed ▶

ADENOMA

THYROID-PARATHYROID

DISEASE PROCESS	CLINICAL, LABORATORY, AND RELATED FINDINGS	ETIOLOGY	ULTRASOUND FINDINGS
Adenoma, *Thyroid* (CONTINUED)			Most are hyperechoic compared to the normal thyroid tissue
			Thin 2- to 3-mm hypoechoic rim or "halo" typically surrounds mass
Carcinoma	"Cold nodule" on nuclear medicine scan (20% of cold nodules are malignant)	Biopsy required to differentiate from adenoma	See each type below
	Has slow growth pattern	Four primary types based on morphology and biologic behavior:	Hemorrhage and cystic degenerative changes appear less frequently than in adenoma
	Clinical presentations include: • Lump in the neck • Hard mass on palpation • History of enlarging goiter • Hoarseness • Pressure symptoms	• Papillary • Follicular • Medullary • Anaplastic	90% have ↑ intra- and perinodular vascularization

DISEASE PROCESS	CLINICAL, LABORATORY, AND RELATED FINDINGS	ETIOLOGY	ULTRASOUND FINDINGS
Anaplastic	• Pain • Satellite lymphadenopathy	Most are mixed papillary-follicular type	Appearance ranges from single nodule to diffuse glandular invasion
	Presents with pressure and neck tenderness	Histologically undifferentiated growth	Solid, hypoechoic mass; may be irregular
	Usually occurs in the seventh or eighth decade of life; affects males more often than females	Extremely malignant	May see metastatic extension to regional lymphatics, appearing as complex, primarily cystic masses adjacent to mass-filled thyroid gland
	Occurs in <15% of thyroid Ca		
	Tumor grows rapidly; early hematogenous and lymphogenous metastasis		
	Fatal		
Follicular	Affects females more often than males ▶	Adenocarcinoma of the thyroid	Usually indistinguishable from benign adenoma ▶

THYROID-PARATHYROID

DISEASE PROCESS	CLINICAL, LABORATORY, AND RELATED FINDINGS	ETIOLOGY	ULTRASOUND FINDINGS
Carcinoma, *Follicular* (*CONTINUED*)	Occurs in 20% of thyroid cancers		Solitary, enlarging, encapsulated nodule
	Microcalcifications are clearly defined on x-ray		Microcalcifications may be imaged
	Causes irregular enlargement of the gland		May appear irregular
	Slow growth pattern		60% have anechoic halo around lesion
	May metastasize hematogenously to lung and bone		
Medullary	Less common; occurs in <10% of all cases	C-cell or parafollicular origin	Appears as solid, hypoechoic, bulky mass
	Hard, palpable mass	Familial distribution with autosomal dominant pattern	May occupy part or all of gland
	Affects serum calcitonin levels		Appears as well-circumscribed lesion without its own capsule

DISEASE PROCESS	CLINICAL, LABORATORY, AND RELATED FINDINGS	ETIOLOGY	ULTRASOUND FINDINGS
	Slow-growing, but metastasizes early lymphogenously and later hematogenously		Granular calcifications appear in 50% of tumors
	Prognosis favorable; 50% 5-year survival rate		
Papillary	Most common type of thyroid cancer (60% of cases)	Wide range of histologic changes from papilliform stroma and follicular elements	Hypoechoic lesion
	Affects children and adults under 40 yrs of age		May range in size from tiny to 10 cm
	More commonly affects females		Microcalcifications may appear as punctate or linear, echogenic foci
	Asymptomatic; painless, palpable lump		

CARCINOMA

DISEASE PROCESS	CLINICAL, LABORATORY, AND RELATED FINDINGS	ETIOLOGY	ULTRASOUND FINDINGS
Cyst			
Simple	Palpable mass or neck swelling	Cystic degeneration of follicular adenoma; may become hemorrhagic spontaneously or as a result of trauma	Well-demarcated, anechoic mass within lobe
	Accounts for the majority of "cold nodules" on radionuclide scan		Smooth walls
			Posterior acoustic enhancement
		The pure thyroid simple cyst is rare	If hemorrhagic, may appear cystic, with low-level echoes, or septated, with reduced acoustic enhancement
			Majority are solitary, <3–4 cm
			Rarely, coarse calcifications at mass periphery are seen

DISEASE PROCESS	CLINICAL, LABORATORY, AND RELATED FINDINGS	ETIOLOGY	ULTRASOUND FINDINGS
Thyroglossal duct	Palpable superficial midline mass superior to isthmus of thyroid	Persistence of thyroglossal duct as a remnant of thyroid gland migration from pharyngeal epithelium	Midline, palpable cystic mass
			Located between hyoid bone and isthmus
	Usually nontender; has rubbery consistency and well-defined margins		Posterior acoustic enhancement
			Rarely larger than 2–3 cm
	Patient may have anterior neck enlargement with pain if cyst is hemorrhagic or infected		If hemorrhagic or infected, appears with internal reflections and dependent debris
Graves' disease (thyrotoxicosis)	Thyromegaly	Thyroid hyperfunction related to production of autoimmune antibodies directed against thyroid causes diffuse cellular hyperplasia	Glands usually enlarged, homogeneous or heterogeneous; hypoechoic compared to normal glands
	$\uparrow T_3$ and T_4		
	Various degrees of exophthalmos		Color Doppler usually shows $\uparrow$ low-impedance vascularity

GRAVES' DISEASE

DISEASE PROCESS	CLINICAL, LABORATORY, AND RELATED FINDINGS	ETIOLOGY	ULTRASOUND FINDINGS
Thyroiditis			
Autoimmune (Hashimoto's)	Most common inflammatory process of thyroid	Infection leading to massive infiltration of lymphocytes into gland	Diffusely enlarged gland
	Occurs predominantly in females between third and fifth decades	Autoimmune disturbance underlying cause	Slightly irregular echo pattern, but primarily hypoechoic compared to adjacent muscles
	Findings include:		Calcifications may occur after inflammation
	• Diffusely enlarged, soft, palpable thyroid		
	• Hoarseness		
	• Neck swelling; may have discomfort		
	Decreased T_3 and T_4 in 50% of patients		

DISEASE PROCESS	CLINICAL, LABORATORY, AND RELATED FINDINGS	ETIOLOGY	ULTRASOUND FINDINGS
Chronic (Reidel's)	Affects women more often than men	Chronic, fibrosing inflammatory process	Diffuse enlargement of both lobes and isthmus
	Usually occurs in the sixth decade of life	Results in asymmetric contraction of the thyroid gland	Heterogeneous echo pattern compared to that of normal gland due to fibrosis and scarring
	Insidious onset	Least common inflammatory process of the thyroid, occurring rarely	
	Patient presents with pressure from adherence of the gland to the trachea and subcutaneous neck tissue		
Subacute (de Quervain's)	Occurs predominantly in females between second and fifth decades of life	Granulomatous inflammation follows viral infection	Diffusely enlarged gland
	Develops acutely or insidiously ▶	Benign	May be asymmetric
		Occurs transiently	Discrete areas of increased and decreased echogenicity

THYROIDITIS

THYROID-PARATHYROID

DISEASE PROCESS	CLINICAL, LABORATORY, AND RELATED FINDINGS	ETIOLOGY	ULTRASOUND FINDINGS
Thyroiditis, *Subacute* (*de Quervain's*) (*CONTINUED*)	Painful swelling of thyroid		
	Fever		
	Gland palpably enlarged either diffusely or focally		
	Increaed T_3 and T_4 in 50% of patients		
	Normal WBC count		
	Usually remits spontaneously		

LIST OF SYMBOLS AND ABBREVIATIONS

SYMBOLS

↑↓	increase, decrease (more than one arrow = marked increase or decrease)
(+)	positive test results
2°	secondary

ABBREVIATIONS

A

AC	abdominal circumference
ACE	acetylcholinesterase
AFI	amniotic fluid volume index
AFP	alpha-fetoprotein
AIDS	acquired immunodeficiency syndrome
ALP	alkaline phosphatase
ALT	alanine aminotransferase (*see* SGPT)
AP	anterior/posterior
APKD	adult polycystic kidney disease
AST	aspartate aminotransferase (*see* SGOT)

B

BCP	birth control pill
BPD	biparietal diameter
BUN	blood urea nitrogen

C

Ca	cancer
CBD	common bile duct
CHD	common hepatic duct
CHF	congestive heart failure
CMV	cytomegalovirus

CNS	central nervous system
CRL	crown-rump length
CSF	cerebrospinal fluid
CSP	cava septum pellucidum
CT	computed tomography
CV	cardiovascular

D

DHEAS	dehydroepiandrosterone sulfate
DISIDA	diisopropyl-iminodi-acetic acid (nuclear medicine)
DNA	deoxyribonucleic acid
Dx	diagnosis

E

EGA	estimated gestational age
EHM	embryonic heart motion
EM	embryonic motion
ETOH	alcohol

F

FHM	fetal heart motion (+++ = heart motion present; – – – = heart motion absent)
FHT	fetal heart tone
FL	femur length
FSH	follicle-stimulating hormone

G

GB	gallbladder
GFR	glomerular filtration rate
GI	gastrointestinal
GU	genitourinary

H

HC	head circumference
hCG	human chorionic gonadotropin

β**-hCG**	human chorionic gonadotropin in beta subunit
HRT	hormone replacement therapy
HTN	hypertension
Hx	history

I

ICH	intracranial hemorrhage
IPH	intraparenchymal hemorrhage
IRDS	infant respiratory distress syndrome
IUD	intrauterine device (contraceptive)
IUGR	intrauterine growth restriction
IUP	intrauterine pregnancy
IVC	inferior vena cava
IVH	intraventricular hemorrhage
IVP	intravenous pyelogram
IVS	intraventricular septum

K

| **KUB** | kidney ureter bladder |

L

LDH	lactate dehydrogenase
LFT	liver function test
LH	luteinizing hormone
LQ	lower quadrant
L/S ratio	lecithin-sphingomyelin ratio
LUQ	left upper quadrant
LV	left ventricle
LVOT	left ventricular outflow tract
LVR	lateral ventricular ratio

M

| **MHz** | megahertz |
| **mIU** | milli-international unit |

MMS	multiple marker screen
MSAFP	maternal serum alpha-fetoprotein

N

NPO	non per os (*L.* nothing through the mouth)
N/V	nausea and vomiting

P

Pap	Papanicolaou smear (or test)
PID	pelvic inflammatory disease
PMB	postmenopausal bleeding
PMN	polymorphonuclear neutrophils
PO$_2$	partial pressure of oxygen
PROM	premature rupture of membrane
PSA	prostatic specific antigen
PV	portal vein

R

RBC	red blood cells
Rh	Rhesus blood factor
RI	resistive index
RLQ	right lower quadrant
RUQ	right upper quadrant
RV	right ventricle
RVOT	right ventricular outflow tract
Rx	treatment

S

S/D ratio	systolic to diastolic ratio
SEH	subependymal hemorrhage
SGOT	serum glutamic-oxaloacetic transaminase (*see* AST)
SGPT	serum glutamate-pyruvate transaminase (*see* ALT)
SLE	systemic lupus erythematosus

SOB	shortness of breath
SV	splenic vein

T

T_3	triiodothyronine
T_4	thyroxine
TB	tuberculosis
TE fistula	tracheal esophageal fistula
TORCH	toxoplasmosis, other (viruses), rubella, cytomegalovirus, herpes (simplex viruses)
Triple screen (MMS)	MSAFP, unconjugated estriol, hCG

U

U/S	ultrasound
UTI	urinary tract infection

V

V-P shunting	ventriculo-peritoneal shunting
VSD	ventral septal defect

W

WBC	white blood cells

X

XX	normal female chromosome type (re: genetics)
XXY	aneuploidy with extra X chromosome (re: genetics)
XY	normal male chromosome type (re: genetics)

SUGGESTED ADDITIONAL READING

BOOKS

Barnes RW, Bergman RT, Hadley HL, et al: Urology, 2nd ed. New York, Medical Examination Publishing, 1974

Beeson P, McDermott W: Textbook of Medicine. Philadelphia, WB Saunders, 1979

Bell WE: Neurologic Infections in Children. Philadelphia, WB Saunders, 1981

Berman MC, Cohen HL: Diagnostic Medical Sonography A Guide to Clinical Practice: Obstetrics and Gynecology, 2nd ed. Philadelphia, Lippincott-Raven, 1997

Callen P: Ultrasonography in Obstetrics and Gynecology, 2nd ed. Philadelphia, WB Saunders, 1988

Connor J, Ferguson-Smith MA: Essential Medical Genetics, 3rd ed. London, Blackwell Scientific Publications, 1991

Copstead LC: Perspectives on Pathophysiology. Philadelphia, WB Saunders, 1995

Ferrucci JT: Radiology Diagnosis Imaging Intervention. Philadelphia, JB Lippincott, 1988

Fleischer A, Manning FA, Jeanty P, et al: Sonography in Obstetrics and Gynecology: Principles and Practice, 5th ed. Stamford, CT, Appleton and Lange, 1996

Gates G: Atlas of Abdominal Ultrasonography in Children. New York, Churchill Livingstone, 1978

Hacker N, Moore J: Essentials of Obstetrics and Gynecology. Philadelphia, WB Saunders, 1986

Hagen-Ansert S: Textbook of Diagnostic Ultrasonography, 3rd ed. St. Louis, CV Mosby, 1988

Hayden C, Swischuk L: Pediatric Ultrasonography. Baltimore, Williams & Wilkins, 1987

Holleb A, Fink D, Murphy G: American Cancer Society Textbook of Clinical Oncology. Atlanta, American Cancer Society, 1991

Jeffrey RB, Ralls PW: Sonography of the Abdomen. New York, Raven Press, 1995

Kawamura D: Abdomen Diagnostic Medical Sonography, A Guide to Clinical Practice. Vol. III. Philadelphia, JB Lippincott, 1991

Kelley V: Practice of Pediatrics, vols. 2 and 5. New York, Harper & Row, 1986

Klaus MH, Fanoroff AA: Care of the High Risk Neonate. Philadelphia, WB Saunders, 1979

Kumer V, Cotran RS, Robbins SL: Basic Pathology, 5th ed. Philadelphia, WB Saunders, 1992

Leech RW, Brumback RA: Hydrocephalus, Current Clinical Concepts. St. Louis, Mosby Yearbook, 1991

Maertens P: Congenital brain pathology. In: Teagler CH, Babikian VL, Gomez CR (eds): Neurosonology. St. Louis, Mosby, 1996

Marshall FF: Urologic Complications, Medical and Surgical, Adult and Pediatric. Chicago, Year Book Medical Publishers, 1986

McCance K, Heather S: Pathophysiology, The Biological Basis for Disease in Adults and Children. St. Louis, CV Mosby, 1990

Meyers M: Dynamic Radiology of the Abdomen: Normal and Pathologic Anatomy. New York, Springer-Verlag, 1976

Moore KL: Clinically Oriented Anatomy, 2nd ed. Baltimore, Williams & Wilkins, 1985

Murphy G: Medical Affairs, vol. III, no. 8. Atlanta, American Cancer Society, 1991

Orrison W: Introduction to Neuro-Imaging. Boston, Little, Brown, 1989

Peterson RO: Urologic Pathology. Philadelphia, JB Lippincott, 1986

Price SA, Wilson LM: Pathophysiology—Clinical Concepts of Disease Process, 3rd ed. New York, McGraw-Hill, 1986

Resnick MI, Sanders RC: Ultrasound in Urology, 2nd ed. Baltimore, Williams & Wilkins, 1984

Robbins S: Pathological Basis of Disease, 3rd ed. Philadelphia, WB Saunders, 1984

Rumack C, Johnson ML: Perinatal and Infant Brain Imaging: Role of Ultrasound and Computed Tomography. Chicago, Year Book Medical Publishers, 1985

Rumack C, Wilson S, Charbonneau JW: Diagnostic Ultrasound, vols. I and II. St. Louis, Mosby Yearbook, 1991

Saltzman RL, Jordan MC: Viral infections. In: Burrow GN, Ferris TF, eds: Medical Complications During Pregnancy, 3rd ed. Philadelphia, WB Saunders, 1988

Sanders R: Clinical Sonography—A Practical Guide. Boston, Little, Brown, 1984

Sandler M, Patton J, Partain C: Thyroid and Parathyroid Imaging. Norwalk, CT, Appleton-Century-Crofts, 1986

Sarti D: Diagnostic Ultrasound, Text and Cases, 2nd ed. Chicago, Year Book Medical Publishers, 1987

Saverbrei EE, Nguyen KT, Nolan RL: A Practical Guide to Ultrasound in Obstetrics and Gynecology. New York, Raven Press, 1987

Skolnick ML: Real Time Ultrasound Imaging in the Abdomen. New York, Springer-Verlag, 1981

Spence A, Mason A: Human Anatomy and Physiology, 2nd ed. Menlo Park, CA, Cummings, 1983

Taylor KJ: Atlas of Ultrasonography, 2nd ed. New York, Churchill Livingstone, 1985

Teele R, Share J: Ultrasonography of Infants and Children. Philadelphia, WB Saunders, 1991

Timor-Tritsch I, Monteagudo A, Cohen H: Ultrasonography of the Prenatal and Neonatal Brain. Stamford, CT, Appleton and Lange, 1996

Truemper EJ, Fischer A: Transcranial Doppler sonography: Diagnosis and pathology. In: Teagler CH, Babikian VL, Gomez CR (eds): Neurosonology. St. Louis, Mosby, 1996

Wallach J: Interpretation of Diagnostic Tests. Boston, Little, Brown, 1979

Walter J: Pathology of Human Disease. Philadelphia, Lea & Febiger, 1989

Walter JB: An Introduction to the Principles of Disease, 2nd ed. Philadelphia, WB Saunders, 1982

Warkany J, Lemire RJ, Cohen NM: Mental Retardation and Congenital Malformations of the Central Nervous System. Chicago, Year Book Medical Publishers, 1981

Yiu-Chiu US, Chiu LC: Atlas of Obstetrical Ultrasonography. Baltimore, University Park Press, 1982

JOURNAL ARTICLES

Adler DD, Samuels BI, Bowerman RA, et al: Sonographic spectrum of focal splenic lesions. JDMS 2:315–320, 1986

Arinbuster D: Prostate-specific antigen: Biochemistry, analytical methods, and clinical applications. Clin Chem 39(2): 181–195, 1993

Atwell J, Levick P: Congenital hypertrophic pyloric stenosis associated anomalies in the genitourinary tract. J Pediatr Surg 16:1029–1031, 1981

Banner MP, Pollack HM, Chatten J, et al: Multilocular renal cysts: Radiologic pathologic correlation. AJR 132:656–658, 1979

Baun J: Neonatal intracranial hemorrhage. JDMS 7:120–131, 1991

Bennett T, Burlbow J, Drake C, et al: Diagnosis of ectopic cordis at 12 weeks gestation using transabdominal ultrasonography with color flow Doppler. JUM 10:695–696, 1991

Benson C, Doubilet P, Richie J: Sonography of the male genital tract. AJR 153:705–713, 1989

Brkljacic B, Sabljar-Matovinovic M, Putarek K, et al: Renal vascular resistance in autosomal dominant polycystic kidney disease: Evaluation with color Doppler ultrasound. Acta Radiol 38(5):840–846, 1997

Brooke J, Laing F, Lewis F: Acute appendicitis; high resolution real-time US findings. Radiology 163:11–14, 1987

Burstein J, Papile LJ, Burstein R: Intraventricular hemorrhage and hydrocephalus in premature neonates: A prospective study with CT. AJR 132:631–635, 1979

Casola G, Schleble W, Leopold G: Neuroblastoma metastatic to the testis: Ultrasonographic screening as an aid to clinical staging. Radiology 151:475–476, 1984

Comstock CH, Culp D, Gonzales J, et al: Agenesis of the corpus callosum in the fetus: Its evolution and significance. JUM 4:613, 1985

David E, van Kaick G, Ikinger U, et al: Detection of neoplastic lymph node involvement in retroperitoneal space. Radiology 148:343, 1983 (Abstract)

Elejalde BR, de Elejalde MMd, Acuna JM, et al: Trisomy 21 prospective study of the ultrasonographic phenotypic characteristics. The Fetus 1(5):7580(1–7), 1991

Eliezer S, Ester F, Ehud W, et al: Fetal splenomegaly ultrasound diagnosis of cytomegalovirus infection: A case report. JCU 12:520–521, 1984

Fong K, Rahmani MR, Rose TH, et al: Fetal renal cystic disease: Sonographic-pathologic correlation. AJR 146:767–773, 1986

Gaines PA, Sampson MA: The prevalence and characterization of simple hepatic cysts by ultrasound exam. Br J Radiol 62:335–337, 1989

Gibney R, Hendin A, Cooperberg P: Sonographically detected hepatic hemangioma: Absence of change over time. AJR 149:953–957, 1987

Gore RM, Callen PW, Filly RA: Displaced retroperitoneal fat: Sonographic guide to right upper quadrant mass localization. Radiology 142:701, 1982

Grant EG: Sonography of the premature brain: Intracranial hemorrhage and periventricular leukomalacia. Neuroradiology 28:476–490, 1986

Grossman H, Rosenberg ER, Bowie JD, et al: Review: Sonographic diagnosis of renal cystic disease. AJR 140:81–85, 1983

Guzzetta F, et al: Periventricular intraparenchymal echodensities in the premature newborn: Critical determinant of neurologic outcome. Pediatrics 78:995–1006, 1986

Haller JO, Cohen HL: Hypertrophic pyloric stenosis: Diagnosis using ultrasound. Radiology 161:335–339, 1986

Han B, Babcock D, Gelfand M: Choledochal cyst with bile duct dilatation: Sonography and ^{99m}TcIDA cholescintigraphy. AJR 136:1075–1079, 1981

Hayashi N, Konishi J, Yonekure Y, et al: Sonography of Hashimoto's thyroiditis. JCU 14:123–126, 1986

Hayden CK Jr, Swischuk LE, Lobe TE, et al: Ultrasound: The definitive imaging modality in pyloric stenosis. Radiographics 4(3):517–530, 1984

Hedgcock MW Jr, Hricak H: Critical decisions in imaging renal masses. Applied Radiology 6:142–144, 1986

Hertzberg B, Burger, PC, Bowie JD, et al: Sonographic characteristics of small cerebral blood vessels. An in vivo and postmortem study. JUM 9:697–703, 1990

Hertzberg B, Kurtz A, Wapner R: Gestational trophoblastic disease with co-existent normal fetus: Evaluation by ultrasound-guided chorionic villus samples. JUM 5:467–469, 1986

Hilpert P, Kurtz A: Prenatal diagnosis of agenesis of the corpus callosum using endovaginal ultrasound. JUM 9:363–365, 1990

Hiton SVW, Leopold G, Olson LK, et al: Real time breast sonography: Application in 300 consecutive patients. AJR 147:479–486, 1986

Jaffe R: Meckel syndrome. The Fetus 1(5);7598:1–3, 1991

Koontz W, Shaw L, Lavery JP: Antenatal sonographic appearance of Beckwith-Wiedemann syndrome. JCU 14:57–59, 1986

Kurjak A, Zalud I, Schulman H: Ectopic pregnancy: Transvaginal flow in questionable adnexa. JUM 10:685–689, 1991

Lyons E: Early pregnancy loss by endovaginal sonography (EVS). American Institute of Ultrasound in Medicine *State of the Art Ob/Gyn Imaging Course.* San Diego, March 6, 1992

Magill HL, Tonkin ILD, Bada H, et al: Advantages of coronal ultrasound in evaluation of neonatal retroperitoneum. Radiology 151:823, 1984 (Abstract)

Mailloux G, Bertrand M, Stampfler R, et al: Computed tomography in the evaluation of congenital toxoplasmosis. J Comput Assist Tomogr 4:326–329, 1980

Marchal G, Gelin J, Verbeker E, et al: High resolution real-time sonography of the adrenal glands: A routine examination? JUM 5:65–68, 1986

Masdeu J, Dobben G, Azar-Kia B: Dandy–Walker syndrome studied by computed tomography and pneumoencephalography. Radiology 147:109–114, 1983

Murray JC, Johnson JA, Bird TD: Dandy–Walker malformation: Etiologic heterogeneity and empiric recurrence risks. Clin Genet 28:272–283, 1985

Naidich TP, Yousef Zadah DK, Gusnard DA: Part II. The neonatal head, Sonography of the normal neonatal head supratentorial structures: State of the art imaging. Neuroradiology 28:408–427, 1986

Nomura G, Kinoshita E, Yamagata Y, et al: Usefulness of renal ultrasonography for assessment of severity and course of acute tubular necroses. JCU 12:135–139, 1984

Norman A, Brenbridge AG, Buschi AJ, et al: Renal emphysema of the transplanted kidney: Sonographic appearance. AJR 132:656–658, 1979

Norton K, Rabinowitz JG: Ultrasonic imaging of abdominal masses in neonates. Appl Radiol 6:81–100, 1986

Nyberg DA, Cyr DR, Mack LA, et al: The Dandy–Walker malformation: Prenatal sonographic diagnosis and its clinical significance. JUM 7:65–71, 1988

Parulekar S: Sonography of the normal fetal bowel. JNM 10:211–220, 1991

Pasto ME, Kurtz AB: Part I. Fetal neurosonographic ultrasonography of the normal fetal brain. Neuroradiology 28:380–385, 1986

Patriquin H, Lafortune M, Fliatraut D: Urinary milk of calcium in children and adults: Use of gravity dependent sonography. AJR 144:407–413, 1985

Pavone P, Di Cesare E, Di Renzi P, et al: Abdominal aortic aneurysm evaluation: Comparison of US, CT, MRI, and angiography. MRI Imaging 8:199–204, 1990

Potter JL, Sullivan BM, Flournoy JG, et al: Emphysema in the renal allograft. Radiology 155:51–52, 1985

Puylart J: Acute appendicitis: US evaluation using graded compression. Radiology 158:355–360, 1986

Sample F: A new technique for the evaluation of the adrenal gland with gray scale ultrasonography. Radiology 124: 463–469, 1977

Satin A, Twickler D, Wendel JG: Congenital syphilis associated with dilation of fetal small bowel. A case report. JUM 11:49–52, 1992

Schölmerech J, Volk BA: Differential diagnosis of anechoic/ hypoechoic lesions in the abdomen detected by ultrasound. JCU 14:339–353, 1986

Sherer DM, Abramowicz JS, Woods JR: Pleural effusion, bilateral transient. The Fetus 1(4);7488:1–3, 1991

Sitzman J, Imbembo A: Splenic complications of a pancake pseudocyst. Am J Surg 147:191–196, 1984

Spirit BA, Gordon LP, Cohen WN, et al: Antenatal diagnosis of chorioangioma of placenta. AJR 135:1273, 1991

Sudakoff G, Mitchell D, Stanley C, et al: Frontal periventricular cysts on the first day of life. A one-year clinical follow-up and its significance. JUM 10:25–30, 1991

Tanaka S, Kitamura T, Fujita M, et al: Color Doppler flow imaging of liver tumors. AJR 154:509–514, 1990

Teefey SA, Baron RL, Bigler SA: Sonography of the gallbladder: Significance of striated (layered) thickening of the gallbladder wall. AJR 156:945–947, 1991

Townsend RR, Laing FC, Jeffrey RB: Placenta abruption associated with cocaine abuse. AJR 150:1339–1340, 1988

Wheeler TC, Dao A, Jeanty P: Hydranencephaly. The Fetus 1(2);7423:1–4, 1991

Yashiro N, Yoshida H, Araki T: Bilateral "milk of calcium" renal cysts: CT findings. J Comput Assist Tomogr 9:199–200, 1985

Yucel E, Fillmore D, Knox T, Waltman A: Sonographic measurement of abdominal aortic diameter: Interobserver variability. JUM 10:681–683, 1991